The Hospital Power Equilibrium

The Johns Hopkins Series in Contemporary Medicine and Public Health

Consulting Editors

Samuel H. Boyer IV, M.D.
Gareth M. Green, M.D., M.P.H.
Richard T. Johnson, M.D.
Paul R. McHugh, M.D.
Edmond A. Murphy, M.D.
Albert H. Owens, Jr., M.D.
Jerry L. Spivak, M.D.
Barbara Starfield, M.D., M.P.H.

David W. Young
Richard B. Saltman

The Hospital Power Equilibrium
Physician Behavior and Cost Control

The Johns Hopkins University Press

Baltimore and London

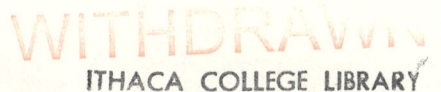

©1985 The Johns Hopkins University Press
All rights reserved
Printed in the United States of America

The Johns Hopkins University Press,
701 West 40th Street, Baltimore, Maryland 21211
The Johns Hopkins Press Ltd, London

The paper in this book is acid-free and meets the
guidelines for permanence and durability of the
Committee on Production Guidelines for Book
Longevity of the Council on Library Resources.

Library of Congress Cataloging in Publication Data

Young, David W.
  The hospital power equilibrium.

  (The Johns Hopkins series in contemporary medicine
and public health)
  Bibliography: p.
  Includes index.
  1. Hospitals—Sociological aspects. 2. Power (Social
sciences) 3. Physicians—Psychology. 4. Hospitals—
Staff—Psychology. 5. Hospital care—Cost control.
6. Hospitals—United States—Sociological aspects—
Case studies. 7. Physicians—United States—
Psychology—Case studies. 8. Hospitals—
United States—Staff—Psychology—Case studies.
I. Saltman, Richard B. II. Title. III. Series.
[DNLM: 1. Cost Control. 2. Decision Making.
3. Economics, Hospital—United States. 4. Hospital
Administration—economics—United States. 5. Role.
WX 157 Y69h]
RA965.Y68   1985   361.1'1   85-9820
ISBN 0-8018-2794-9 (alk. paper)

To
Michela and Christian
Denise and Julian

Contents

Acknowledgments   ix

Part 1   The Scope of the Problem

1   The Cost Containment Challenge   3
   Implications of Market-Based Proposals   3
   The Failure of Regulation   13
   A Misconception of the Market   17
   The Challenge to Policymakers   19

2   The Hospital Power Equilibrium: A Theoretical Framework   21
   Theories of Hospital Decision Making   21
   Gaps in the Theory   24
   The Theory of Power Equilibrium   25
   Occupational Strategies in the Hospital   28
   The Power Equilibrium in the Hospital   31
   Cost Containment and the Power Equilibrium   35

3   Behavioral Incentives in the Hospital Power Equilibrium   39
   The Impetus toward Institutional Growth   39
   Incentives for Physicians   42
   Incentives for Administrators   46
   Incentives for Other Occupational Groups   48
   Consequences of Group Behavioral Incentives   49
   Implications for Cost Containment   52

Part 2   The Case Studies

4   The Decision-Making Structure at Peninsula Community Hospital   57
   The Setting   57
   Budget Structure   59
   Interactions between Physicians and Administrators   59
   Interactions within the Medical Staff   63
   Interactions between Medical Staff and Support Staff   65
   Medical Staff Cost Containment Issues   67
   Conclusions   71

5   The Decision-Making Structure at Oak Memorial Medical Center   72
   The Setting   72
   Budget Structure   73
   Interactions between Physicians and Administrators   73
   Interactions within the Administration   78
   Interactions within the Medical Staff   79

viii   *Contents*

        Interactions between Medical Staff and Support Staff   86
        Conclusions   88

6   Programmatic Decision Making at Peninsula
    Community Hospital   89
        Decision-Making Criteria   89
        Program Initiatives   92
        Summary   103

7   Programmatic Decision Making at Oak Memorial
    Medical Center   104
        Senior Management's Perspective   104
        Middle Management's Perspective   105
        Service Chiefs' Perspective   110
        The Role of Fiscal Affairs   117
        Summary   119

8   An Analysis of the Two Power Equilibria   120
        Methodological Questions   120
        Theoretical Implications of the Case Studies   121
        Cost Containment Issues   129
        Implications for Health Policy and Management   138

Part 3   Cost Containment, Public Policy, and the
            Hospital Power Equilibrium

9   The Need for Centralized Management Control Systems   143
        Cost Sharing and Hospital-Based Programs   143
        Cost Containment and Management Control Systems   144
        Centralized versus Decentralized Management
            Control Systems   147
        Structural Failures of Existing Reimbursement Systems   153
        Summary   157

10   Realigning Regulatory Control   158
        The Management Control Structure   158
        The Management Control Process   163
        Integrating Physicians into Hospital Management   167
        Establishing Effective Hospital Top Management   169
        Advantages of a Matrix-Based Control System   172
        Conclusions   173

Notes   175

References   185

Index   195

Acknowledgments

Like many works of this sort, this book has a rather long history. During the five years over which it has evolved, we have incurred an enormous number of intellectual and other debts, and are delighted to have an opportunity to thank all those individuals and organizations that have given so freely of their time and resources.

First, we owe a major obligation to the two hospitals in which we conducted our research. It is not easy for an organization to open its doors to investigators engaged in exploratory research, nor is it easy to be candid about some of the very sensitive issues we were raising. Since the identities of the organizations are disguised, we cannot thank by name the various administrators, physicians, nurses, and others who made themselves available to us and shared their views. Nevertheless, we are most grateful to everyone involved.

The research would not have been possible without the financial support provided by several foundations and other sources. Grants to the Department of Health Policy and Management at the Harvard School of Public Health from the Kellogg Foundation and the Kaiser Family Foundation allowed us to conduct our interviews and prepare some of the early portions of the manuscript. Sabbatical funds from the Harvard School of Public Health, a grant from the Milton Fund of the Harvard Medical School, and a Curriculum Development grant from the Pew Memorial Trust funded completion of the manuscript. We are most appreciative of this support and hope the sponsors will feel that their funding decisions were wise ones.

The Department of Health Policy and Management and the School of Public Health provided us with an intellectually stimulating base from which to conduct our research. Moreover, colleagues at the school and elsewhere provided invaluable feedback on our efforts. Sometimes this feedback came in a large-group format, as when we presented our preliminary findings at departmental colloquia attended by both faculty and students, and sometimes it was individual. In particular, we would like to single out Jonathan Brown, Martin Chin, Rose Laub Coser, Harvey Fineberg, Alfred Gelhorn, Howard Hiatt, Nancy Kane, Harry Marks, Frederick Mosteller, William Stason, and Alan Sheldon, all of whom read portions of the manuscript and made comments that helped us to clarify and strengthen our arguments. Anders Richter of the Johns Hopkins University Press and Theodore Marmor of Yale University, who read the completed manuscript, provided suggestions and support as we revised the manuscript into final form.

Several journals in which we have published portions of our overall argument were most generous in allowing us to reproduce material. Portions of the manuscript have appeared in "The Hospital Power Equilibrium: An Alternative View of the Cost Containment Dilemma," *Journal of Health Politics, Policy and Law* 6 (1981): 391–418 (part of chap. 1, chap. 2); "Medical Practice, Case Mix and Cost Containment: A New Role for the Attending Physician," *Journal of the American Medical Association* 247 (1982): 801–5, copyright 1982, American Medical Association (part of chap. 10); "Preventive Medicine for Hospital Costs," *Harvard Business Review* 61 (1983): 126–34, copyright 1983 by the President and Fellows of Harvard College (part of chap. 10); "Hospital Cost Containment and the Quest for Institutional Growth: A Behavioral Analysis," *Journal of Public Health Policy* 4 (1983): 313–34 (part of chap. 3); and "Prospective Reimbursement and the Hospital Power Equilibrium: A Matrix-Based Management Control System," *Inquiry* 20 (1983): 20–33 (parts of chaps. 9 and 10). Several small segments also appear in David Young's *Financial Control in Health Care* (Homewood, Illinois: Dow-Jones-Irwin, 1984).

We also would like to express our appreciation to Alice M. Bennett, our copy editor, and to the rather large number of secretarial and administrative staff members who assisted us in preparing the manuscript at various stages in its development. Regina Anderson, Lynette Coleman, Mary Corcoran, Deborah Harris, Deborah Katz, Cathrine Lowndes, Matara Malone, Katy Morakis, Kathleen O'Brien, Jaylyn Olivo, of the Harvard School of Public Health, and the staff of the Mulberry Studio in Cambridge, Massachusetts, were all involved at one time or another in the saga.

Finally, our wives and children provided encouragement, support, and perspective during what were occasionally very trying times in the project's five-year life cycle.

We hope this list has reaffirmed that a research project of this sort is anything but an individual effort. Nevertheless, despite all the assistance, advice, criticism, suggestions, and support we received, it is with both pleasure and relief that we accept full responsibility for the final product.

The Hospital Power Equilibrium

PART 1
The Scope of the Problem

The rapid and continuing growth of national health expenditures has created a dilemma for federal and state health policymakers. On the one hand, as health costs consume an ever greater share of public budgets, policy framers face insistent demands to develop and institute stringent cost containment programs. Yet these same cost increases convincingly demonstrate that existing policy tools and procedures cannot adequately separate necessary from unnecessary patient-care expenditures. Health policymakers thus find themselves boxed into a politically uncomfortable corner. Confronted with a financially unsustainable demand on public funds yet lacking sufficiently well targeted cost containment tools, their only apparent alternative is to make medically and socially unacceptable reductions in the care of publicly funded patients.

Federal and state policymakers are also under pressure from the private side of the health care system, particularly from health insurance carriers and large corporate employers. Many Blue Cross plans, for example, faced with growing resistance to higher premiums, have introduced various administrative cost containment mechanisms. The fragmented structure of most state reimbursement systems, however, simply encourages hospitals to allocate any costs disallowed by Blue Cross to commercially insured or charge-paying patients. Commercial carriers, in turn, have become increasingly reluctant to accept such cost shifting and have begun to insist that policymakers provide them with relief.

Employers, for whom these dilemmas translate into higher and higher health insurance premiums, also have begun to raise their voices in concern. When large employers join with their health insurance carriers to demand remedial legislation, as they did recently in Massachusetts (Iglehardt 1982; Caper and Blumenthal 1983; Kinzer 1983), the pressure on policymakers demands action of some sort, regardless of its implications for either patients or providers. Yet the consequences for both, but particularly for publicly funded patients, can become overwhelming.

The present degree of policy paralysis is illustrated by the increasing reliance of both public and private insurers on patient cost sharing mechanisms. In tacit acknowledgment that the nation's health care system, as now organized, cannot deliver adequate services at acceptable cost, advocates of cost sharing seek an immediate reduction in the volume of care the system provides. Unfortunately, this market-based approach is not capable of distributing service reductions evenly across all types of patients, nor will it focus only upon individuals who currently receive excessive care. On the contrary, its market character dictates that service reductions will be borne disproportionately by those with limited financial resources, but who often have substantially greater medical needs: the poor, the elderly, and the chronically ill.

The cost containment dilemma has been further complicated by Medicare's introduction, in October 1983, of a per admission form of reimbursement for hospitals, relying on diagnosis-related groups (DRGs). This has totally changed the incentives for providers of inpatient hospital care. Rather than being reimbursed on a per diem basis for the costs they incur, hospitals now receive a flat rate for each Medicare patient admitted, based on the individual's diagnosis, and are thus financially motivated to spend less than that amount. Whether this incentive system will lower the quality of care received by Medicare patients remains to be seen, but it is already clear that many hospitals throughout the country are encountering new forms of organizational stress as physicians and administrators confront each other over the balance between clinical and financial concerns.

This book has been written in response to many of these issues, but in particular to the cost containment dilemmas faced by hospitals and their attending physicians. Our principal intent is to develop a new set of integrated policy and management tools that can restrain inpatient hospital costs without denying needed care, particularly to the most vulnerable segments of the nation's population. In large part the book is based on the contention that past cost containment and regulatory programs have not been designed to control a key cost-generating factor in the health care system: the attending physician. By focusing on the general issue of inpatient hospital care, which consumes nearly 45 percent of the nation's health budget, we are able to examine the area of the health care system that has perhaps the highest potential for cost savings.

In this first part, we outline the current policy dilemma in the health care sector and present an alternative theoretical framework for hospital behavior. Chapter 1 spells out the cost containment challenge in greater detail. In chapter 2 we explore the structure of decision making within nonprofit, acute-care hospitals and suggest an alternative theory of hospital behavior based on what we term "the hospital power equilibrium." We then draw upon this theory in chapter 3 to examine the incentives that motivate specific occupational groups within the hospital, particularly physicians and administrators, and assess the long-term implications of these incentives for overall institutional behavior. This, then, sets the stage both for the empirical findings discussed in part 2 and for the new policy tools we propose in part 3.

CHAPTER 1
The Cost Containment Challenge

The broad outline of the health care cost problem in the United States is well known. As table 1 indicates, health care expenditures have increased at a consistently high rate over the past twenty years, outpacing nearly every other indicator in the consumer price index. During the fifteen years from 1967 (when Medicare and Medicaid came into being) to 1982 (when the worst economic downturn since the 1930s took hold), the absolute rate of annual health expenditure increase remained in double-digit figures, with total consumption rising to 10.5 percent of the gross national product (GNP).[1] Similarly, although preliminary 1983 and 1984 figures indicated a dramatic decrease in health care inflation to well below 10 percent, health-related consumption still increased at approximately twice the overall economy's inflation rate — a trend that demonstrates continued increase in the share of national income devoted to health care and portends rapid future growth if the general inflation rate should rise. These figures are arguably the highest in the world for an economically stable industrialized nation. In Western Europe and Asia, only Sweden spends a full 10 percent of its GNP on health care, but the Swedes receive a far more comprehensive set of benefits for this expenditure than do most Americans.[2]

Although almost everyone in the United States now recognizes that health care costs cannot continue to spiral upward in this fashion, there is much less agreement on how we can best slow their growth. This lack of consensus exists even though escalating expenditures have dominated health policy debates for more than a decade. With the advent of the Reagan administration in 1980, the fundamental thrust of the debate was altered dramatically. The effort to rationalize expenditures through an interlocking network of government regulation was jettisoned, and emphasis shifted toward various forms of market-style "competition." Since ten years of increasing regulation had failed to modify providers' cost behavior, the administration argued, the necessary fiscal discipline could be achieved only through reliance upon what it termed "market forces." Among the most commonly advanced market-based schemes are increased provider competition and mechanisms to impose greater "cost sharing" on patients when they seek care.

Implications of Market-Based Proposals

The many market-based proposals presented over the past several years all share the common conceptual foundation that patients have been excessively insulated from the cost of the medical services they receive and that

Table 1 Health Care Expenditures: Gross National Product and Consumer Price Index, 1964–83 (in billions of dollars)

Year	Health Expenditures	CPI	GNP	Health Expenditures as Percentage of GNP	Growth Rates Health Expenditures	CPI
1964	35.6	92.9	628.7	5.8	7.6	1.3
1965	41.7	94.5	691.0	6.0	17.1	1.7
1966	42.3	97.2	749.9	5.9	1.4	2.9
1967	48.2	100.0	793.5	6.2	13.9	2.9
1968	53.9	104.2	865.7	6.5	11.8	4.2
1969	59.9	109.8	930.3	6.7	11.1	5.4
1970	74.7	116.3	993.0	7.5	24.7	5.9
1971	83.3	121.3	1,054.9	7.7	11.5	4.3
1972	93.5	125.3	1,158.0	7.9	12.2	3.2
1973	103.2	133.1	1,294.9	7.8	10.4	6.2
1974	116.4	147.7	1,434.0	8.1	12.8	11.0
1975	132.7	161.2	1,549.0	8.6	14.0	9.1
1976	149.7	170.5	1,718.0	8.7	12.8	5.8
1977	169.2	181.5	1,918.0	8.8	13.0	6.5
1978	189.3	195.4	2,164.0	8.8	11.9	7.7
1979	215.0	217.3	2,418.0	8.9	13.6	11.3
1980	249.0	246.8	2,632.0	9.5	15.8	13.5
1981	286.6	272.4	2,954.0	9.8	15.1	10.4
1982	322.4	289.1	3,073.0	10.5	12.5	6.1
1983		297.1 (May)				3.5 (May)

Sources: U.S. Department of Commerce, Bureau of Census, *Statistical Abstract of the United States,* 1966, 1969, 1970, 1974, 1975, 1979, 1980, 1984.

this financial overprotection is a major factor in rising health care costs (Stockman 1981). Proponents of market-based solutions generally suggest some combination of three elements. First, they advocate increased competition among providers, including the relatively unrestrained entry of new providers into the system. Second, they desire increased cost sensitivity among potential recipients of health care services at the time they purchase their health insurance. They would achieve this by eliminating the tax exclusion on employee health care benefits or by issuing vouchers that could be redeemed for health insurance, cash, or some combination of the two, so that the lower one's insurance premium the higher one's cash rebate. Third, they call for increased cost sensitivity among patients at the time they seek or receive health care services. The mechanism used to implement this approach is called "cost sharing" and consists of deductibles and copayments.

Clearly, some combination of all three elements would be necessary to a successful market-based approach. For consumers to have both high-

and low-cost insurance options at the time of purchase, there must be provider competition and alternatives such as health maintenance organizations (HMOs). Moreover, a low-cost option generally incorporates increased cost sharing so that consumers pay part of the cost of care indirectly through premiums and part directly through copayments and deductibles when they receive care.

The central thrust of the market-based approach, then, is cost sharing. Its intent is to make patients less insulated from the cost of care. Thus, argue its supporters, consumers will desire fewer and less expensive services than they do at present, and the inflationary spiral in health care costs will be broken.[3]

These market-based proposals, in particular cost sharing, reflect an extension into the health sphere of a basic economic premise that buyers, when forced to pay the full cost of a seller's services, will be wiser and more careful users of those services. As a result, say the economists, buyers' purchase decisions discipline the price, product quality, and production efficiency of sellers.

Unfortunately, this premise ignores both the intrinsic character of the demand for health services and the complex structure of the health care market itself. As physicians and other health professionals well understand, the relationship between buyer and seller in the provision of health services is anything but bilateral. Instead, medical care, and particularly its most expensive component, inpatient hospital care, is characterized by a complex four-actor relationship, in which A (the patient) is treated by B (the hospital staff) at the behest of C (the attending physician) and paid for by D (the insurance carrier). To presume that patients can discipline hospital staffs and physicians through a market relationship with insurers is to ignore the indirect structure of the relationship, not to mention the highly specialized nature of medical expertise and the life-threatening consequences of inadequate care.

In short, by placing its emphasis upon patients' decisions to *seek* care, cost sharing effectively blames them for financial decisions made by hospitals and physicians in the *provision* of care. Conversely, cost sharing's concentration upon the most peripheral, and least powerful, element in this four-actor relationship means that it will have little, if any, impact on the other forces generating increases in the cost of care.

This faulty economic foundation suggests that reliance upon increased levels of patient cost sharing will not fulfill the expectations of its proponents. On the contrary, far from producing a medically or socially optimal distribution of services in the health sector, this so-called market solution can be expected to interfere substantially with the provision of both adequate care to patients and adequate revenues to providers. We will explore each of these likely consequences in turn.

IMPLICATIONS FOR PATIENTS

As we noted above, a central goal of the cost sharing approach is to tighten the connection between patients' demand for medical services and the cost of delivering those services. More specifically, by imposing a price on patients' decisions to "enter" the health care system, cost sharing programs presumably will deter them from seeking care unnecessarily, and health care costs will fall as a result.

There appears to be little doubt that such a pricing mechanism is effective in reducing the number of primary care visits patients seek. Empirical studies by Roemer et al. (1975), Newhouse et al. (1981), and Brook et al. (1983), among others, have all shown a sharp decrease in primary care visits when copayments and deductibles are imposed. What is less clear, however, is the effect of such an approach on matters of equity, health status, and *overall* health care costs.

Conrad and Marmor (1980) address the equity issue cogently, stating that insurance plans with uniform deductibles or coinsurance rates impose relatively greater burdens on low-income families than on high-income ones. As a result, use of medical services varies not solely with illnesses but also with income (390). Weller and Manga (1983) make essentially the same argument, emphasizing that "user fees" are basically a regressive form of financing that shifts the burden of cost from the public to the private sector and reintroduces financial risks to the sick, which is precisely what publicly financed systems are designed to eliminate (511–12).

In short, it appears that while cost sharing will ration access to care, it will not do so in an equitable fashion. Indeed, it will place a greater economic burden both on low-income families and on individuals who have a proportionately greater need for care, such as the elderly and the chronically ill.

The consequences for health status are not so easy to discern. In what was to be the definitive answer to this issue, the Rand Corporation (Brook et al. 1983) found mixed results. Use of free care in the Rand study, as contrasted with the use of copayments and deductibles, led to an improvement in some measures of health status but not in others. The authors concluded that "although free care did not improve health status across the entire range of measures or income groups examined, it did confer demonstrable benefits for patients with selected conditions that physicians are trained to manage" (1433). More important, however, as the authors themselves acknowledged, no good model of causality was developed: "Precisely how increased use of care led to improvement in some measures of health status and why it did not in others are not yet known" (1433).

A variety of other researchers have addressed the health status issue, albeit somewhat less directly. Mechanic (1980) has noted, for instance, that when patients are forced to decide which conditions merit professional attention, they seek relief for symptoms that cause immediate discomfort rather than for those that may be medically threatening. Conrad and Marmor (1980) point out that cost sharing "might deter people, especially the poor, from seeking necessary care early, thereby adversely affecting health and leading to greater use of services in the long run" (391).

It is this latter effect that results in a blending of health status question with the matter of overall health care costs, particularly when one moves from the short run to the long run. In one of the earliest attempts to look at this relationship between cost sharing and systemwide costs, Roemer et al. (1975) conducted a study of Medicaid patients in California. They found that a one-dollar copayment for a primary care visit sharply reduced the number of such visits, but that the initial savings were more than offset by subsequent increases in hospitalizations for these same patients — hospitalizations that could have been avoided in many instances had patients received adequate and timely primary care. The result was higher financial costs for the system as a whole, not to mention an adverse effect on the health of patients and their families.

Similar concerns about the balance between short-run savings and long-run costs have been raised by Barer et al. (1979, 1982), Beck (1974), Badgley and Smith (1979), Ginzberg (1983a), and others. Ginzberg (1983b) has also pointed out that one of the potential long-term negative effects of cost sharing and other market-based schemes would be an absence of controls over new facility construction, which could easily result in excess system capacity, but with an uneven distribution, so that there would be "pockets" of inadequate health care services. Once again the questions of health status and system costs become intertwined.

The issue of overall system costs has still another twist, however, one central to the basic theme of this book. By examining closely the effects of cost sharing, we can see that the systemwide financial impact is felt in essentially two ways. First, as noted above, if patients defer care, their health may deteriorate so that it costs more to treat them in the long run than it would had they sought timely primary care. Second, it is important to recognize that cost sharing is largely impotent once patients have entered the health care system. At that point, their physician-agents take over and make almost all cost-inducing decisions.

This latter point runs through much of the current literature on cost sharing. Newhouse et al. (1981), describing the results of the Rand study, for example, found that cost sharing provisions had no discernible effect upon the cost of care once patients were hospitalized. Gabel and Monheit (1983) point out that "since patients relinquish much of their consumer sovereignty to their physician-agents, provider incentives are crucial to the determination of health care expenditures" (615). Moore et al. (1983) in reviewing the SAFECO experience, stress that the critical factor for the long-term success of any plan is control of costs once patients have entered the system, and that physicians therefore are involved in the relevant choices. As Weller and Manga (1983) emphasize, "there is little evidence that unnecessary demand has been the main cause of cost escalation (but quite a lot of evidence that it is supplier induced)" (511).

In summary, the structure of the health care market, combined with the nature of patient demand for care, suggests, first, that the practical effect of cost sharing is to ration patients' access to care according to their ability or willingness to pay the out-of-pocket charges for each service rather than according to their *need* for care. As such, it is a financial or psychological impediment to patients' entry into the health care system. Second, the primary effect of increased cost sharing would most likely be on patients' initial decision to seek professional care, not on the costs incurred once they enter the health care system. Third, it encourages self-diagnosis and consequently may be both medically and financially counterproductive. Fourth, as illustrated by the four-actor model of the health care market described above, increased cost sharing by patients can be expected to have little influence on the delivery of unnecessary or inappropriate care by medical providers.

Finally, and of importance to at least *some* policymakers, patients do not *like* the idea of copayments, deductibles, and other cost sharing features. Gabel and Monheit (1983), in assessing employees' response to the Federal Employee Health Benefit Package, found that only 10 percent of the employees were enrolled in an HMO-type organization, and only 13 percent chose a lower-option fee for service indemnity or service plan. They concluded "it may take more than the stimulus from increased consumer cost sharing and reduced tax subsidies to create an environment conducive to competitive provider behavior" (635). Somewhat more emotionally, Snoke (1982) points out that

> people do not buy health care as they do clothes or groceries. They do not want to go to doctors or to hospitals anymore than they want to go to funeral homes. They usually ask for health care because they need it or because they think they need it. It is a rare person who can assess the quality or quantity of care that he or she needs and equate it with the costs. (1030)

Brown (1983) concurs, providing a slightly different perspective:

> A person insures against risks precisely because he does not want to be confronted with such questions of willingness to pay in the unhappy event of illness. He buys health insurance because he does not know what objective conditions (illnesses) may strike; because he does not know exactly how he will

feel about the value of alternative treatments for various objective conditions of various degrees of severity; and because he does not feel capable of deciding and does not want to be forced to decide what the benefit-cost ratios are for various combinations of treatment and illness. Anxiety levels are apt to be too high and the professional expertise of the patient too low to permit him to make rational decisions when an illness strikes. (520-21)

As a consequence, unions and other employee groups can be expected to oppose cost sharing plans, as they have in the past, and even if substantial cost sharing options were available, it appears only individuals who felt they had no financial alternative would select them. Thus the principal result of increased cost sharing would be to further fragment the health care system between the haves and have-nots, impeding access to adequate health care for the most vulnerable segments of our population.

IMPLICATIONS FOR PROVIDERS

The cost sharing strategy yields equally few benefits for the nation's medical providers, particularly hospitals. Indeed, the universalization of high cost sharing forms of health insurance can be expected to deepen the financial difficulties of the nation's acute-care system. Hard-pressed urban hospitals, especially public urban facilities, can expect that increased cost sharing will translate directly into higher bad debt or free care, or both, and that increased use of HMOs will lead to market pressure for pricing many services at or near marginal costs. In fact the latter effect already exists in some areas, and if increased cost sharing raises bad debt and free care levels or succeeds in reducing hospitals' overall service volume, it is likely that many institutions will face additional revenue shortfalls. These three elements combined — marginal cost pricing, higher bad debts and free care, and a reduced patient census — may well force some institutions to increase their charges (to charge payers such as commercial insurance companies) still further so as to cover their fixed costs (those costs associated with a hospital's "readiness to serve" that are present regardless of the number of days of care or other service units provided).

If institutions are successful in raising their present charges still higher in order to offset revenue shortfalls, there will be even greater cross-subsidization among third-party payers than now exists. If they are unsuccessful in this effort, they will need to either seek revenues from other sources (e.g., philanthropy) or close their doors. This will be particularly true for those hospitals that serve a high proportion of Medicare and Medicaid patients and therefore do not have a high charge-paying base.

While one might argue that reducing hospital beds is a necessary step in cost containment (Egdahl 1984), most policy analysts would agree that such reductions should be based on a socially equitable strategic plan, rather than as a consequence of serving lower-income patients. As Cohodes (1983) has suggested, if closings are based solely on revenue shortfalls, we can expect that the resulting reductions in beds and facilities will come precisely in those areas that require more, not fewer, health services.

Unfortunately, this point has become more than just speculation. Many hospitals currently face revenue shortfalls as a result of increased pressures brought on by HMOs, changes in the method of Medicare reimbursement, and in some instances, reimbursement changes for Medicaid patients. Charges of "patient dumping" (private hospitals sending patients who have inadequate insurance to municipal or other public facilities) have become common, and a number of hospitals — particularly those in large metropolitan areas — are on the point of closing their doors. In a recent article in the Chicago *Tribune,* for example, the acting director of the Chicago Health Systems Agency stated, "The hospitals that are in the worst financial shape tend to be those that serve the poor, . . . and they are the ones that are most needed in their communities."[4] A study by Kane (1984) showed a similar pattern in New York City hospitals, and Longo and Chase (1984) suggest that the problem is national in scope. Although most of these financial difficulties are not caused by cost sharing per se, they are in large part the result of market-based pressures. More important, they are the harbinger of the problems hospitals would face under cost sharing schemes, where low-income patients would be unable to meet the deductible and copayment requirements of inpatient hospital care.

If, however, as some market-based proponents argue, the effect of this "industry shakeup" is to restructure the mix of providers, placing greater emphasis on HMOs and other alternative delivery systems, the resulting hospital closings might be quite acceptable. Leaving aside for the moment the critical question emphasized above concerning the *location* of hospitals that remain, what would be the effect of this new provider mix? To answer this we must look at the characteristics of such a system.

Enthoven (1980) has presented an idealized version of the health delivery pattern that would emerge under a competitive market-based system. He would replace the present health insurance system with a multitude of insurer-generated "organized systems of care," structured much like existing HMOs. In Enthoven's scenario, however, all insurer/providers would be required by federal legislation to provide the same minimum level of service, so as to force them to compete for subscribers primarily on the basis of premium price. Hence, under Enthoven's scheme, differences among plan premiums would reflect not cost sharing or restricted service provisions, but rather the higher or lower production efficiencies of different HMOs.

Unfortunately, in a world of imperfect markets, it is highly unlikely that Enthoven's system would function as envisioned. Just as hospitals and physicians now have strong economic incentives to increase services in order to increase revenue, HMOs have a strong incentive to deliver the minimum necessary services in order to decrease costs. To argue, as Enthoven does, that a competitive all-HMO market will ensure the provision of quality care to all individuals is to ignore the reality of these incentive patterns. If HMOs become the universal delivery organizations for health care, each HMO will have a substantial incentive to maximize the number of healthy (and thus less expensive) subscribers on its rolls. Some, if not many, HMOs would seek to avoid enrolling individuals with preexisting medical conditions and to induce expensive subscribers who *have* enrolled to switch to some other HMO. Although Enthoven's plan prevents overt discrimination, obstacles to undesired subscribers can take a number of more subtle forms, including location of treatment facilities, available medical subspecialties, socioeconomic background of the staff, and so forth. Such behavior may appear crass, but it nonetheless is precisely the economically logical incentive that "competition among organized systems of care" would generate.

One must further wonder about the absence of any restriction in Enthoven's plan upon the formation of all-Medicaid HMOs. This facet of his plan is particularly disturbing given the disastrous experience with unscrupulous capitated system operators in the California Medi-Cal (Medicaid) program in the 1970s.[5]

To date, HMO subscribers have been primarily younger, middle class, and employed. In a "truly competitive" all-HMO world, with all the likely cost-sharing regalia, individuals most in need of care could well become the unwanted stepchildren of market pressures to maintain low premium rates. Once again it is quite likely that this group would comprise the poor, the elderly, and the chronically ill.

The final set of providers that would be affected by a shift toward a more market-oriented health care system is the medical professionals, principally physicians. Cost sharing advocates build a significant part of their case around the idea that physicians would be pressured by their cost-conscious patients to deliver more economical health care. The evidence that this would happen, however, is not reassuring.

In the first place, as discussed above, there appear to be no significant financial savings from cost sharing once a patient enters the hospital. This implies that physicians do not alter their hospital ordering patterns as a result of whatever patient pressure exists. Consequently, the savings from physician behavior changes must come from extrahospital activities, but here too the evidence is weak. Conrad and Marmor (1980) argue, for example, that "physicians and other providers who presumably possess adequate information are only indirectly affected by the prices facing consumers" (391). Gabel and Monheit (1983) conclude that "unless insurers change their reimbursement methods so that providers bear some financial risk for their resource decisions, the health care system is likely to retain much of its inherent inefficiency" (615). Moore et al. (1983), in documenting the SAFECO experience, report that mandatory access through a primary care coordinating physician does decrease ambulatory costs by decreasing the percentage of enrollees using services and specialists, but they go on to point out that these savings are a result of the enrollee's behavior, not that of the physician. Sigelman (1983), discussing why competition will not work, stresses the inability of insurers to affect provider behavior, stating that insurers may lack sufficient "market power" to control providers. It is difficult to believe that if *insurers* lack market power with respect to providers, somehow *patients* can have much influence. Finally, it is not even clear that patients will *want* to control the behavior of their physicians. As Snoke (1982) argues, "No one can be expected to pay much attention to deductibles or coinsurance [sic] at a time of a crisis or when in a hospital" (1030).

Physicians, for their part, are not ignorant of the need for cost-conscious behavior. In a recent survey of physicians' attitudes toward cost containment, Taylor and Paranjpe (1984) found that they generally are less resistant to cost containment that some might think. In fact, two of the factors physicians identified as contributing to excessive system costs were ordering more laboratory tests than necessary and unnecessary hospitalizations, both of which quite clearly are under physician control. Even more significant is the fact that 75 percent of the physicians surveyed believed that the duplication of expensive equipment and specialists at nearby hospitals is a factor contributing to high health care costs *and* that discouraging duplication of this sort is both an acceptable and effective means for cost containment. The implication, as Mechanic (1984) has suggested, is the need to modify the role of physicians from being *advocates* of the patient to being *allocators* of limited resources. "In theory, such an approach brings out the best in professional judgement, since those actually providing the care must make the calculations of tradeoffs" (69).

In short, the evidence to date seems to indicate that cost sharing has little effect on physicians once a patient is hospitalized, and that its ability to make them cost conscious in ambulatory settings is questionable. Yet it is clear that physicians recognize the importance of using health resources judiciously and are prepared to do so. As a result, what seems to be called for are not incentives for *patients,* but rather incentives for *physicians* to encourage them to act upon the cost-conscious rather than the cost-incurring aspects of their professional makeup. This brings us to the topic of regulation.

The Failure of Regulation

Although the cost sharing approach generates a series of unacceptable outcomes, it is nonetheless clear that cost sharing proponents' criticisms of existing American regulatory efforts generally are well founded. These efforts, by and large, have had only minimal success in restraining health care costs at either the national or the state level. While the issues surrounding government regulation of health care may appear to be distinctly different from those involved in cost sharing, both approaches make the same dubious assumptions about the structure of decision making within hospitals. In order to more fully understand the common difficulties that have arisen, however, and to pave the way for the new theoretical scenario we present in chapter 2, we need first to briefly explore the nature of hospital regulatory efforts in the United States to date.

The literature on hospital cost containment documents certain standard assumptions about the sources of hospital cost inflation. The responsibility is usually placed upon some combination of the following: the full-scale emergence of third-party payment; the dramatic changes in medical technology and their associated costs; increases in the number and salaries of hospital personnel; fee for service payment plans; increased capital costs associated with service and facility expansion; inefficient production of services within various hospital departments; and the increased cost of goods and services the hospital purchases from outside suppliers.

These diverse assumptions about the rise in hospital costs have in turn generated a variety of regulatory policies aimed at stemming the increases. Although these policies vary in scope and focus as well as in overall effectiveness, they can usefully be grouped into two broad categories. The first consists of mechanisms designed to regulate and control the operating costs of existing hospitals, in hopes of directly reducing the rate of increase in their costs. The second looks to an alternative set of delivery systems that would reduce the overall patient demand for expensive hospital services and thus the hospital's overall share of total health care expenditures.

The regulatory control category encompasses the growing government effort to reduce the rate of hospital cost increases. At both the state and the federal level, there has been an increasing emphasis upon legislative as well as administrative intervention within current hospital operating procedures. The principal changes include the implementation of prospective reimbursement; the control of hospital charges as well as costs; the introduction of case mix as a factor in reimbursement; the establishment of independent state rate-setting boards; the establishment of controls over capital expansion via certificates of need and health systems agencies; the intensification of utilization review via professional standards review organizations (PSROs) and now professional review organizations (PROs); the use of preferred provider organizations (PPOs); and the establishment of "caps" on capital expenditures.[6]

In contrast to the first approach, the second set of cost containment proposals has sought to encourage the development of alternative delivery systems that can provide nonacute care outside the hospital in less expensive institutional or home settings. Such policies and policy proposals emphasize delivery vehicles such as health maintenance organizations, hospital outpatient care, freestanding surgery and emergency centers, neighborhood health clinics, nursing homes, and home care services.[7] The argument is that these new institutional forms can reduce or eliminate the hospitalization a patient might otherwise require. This result is achieved through a combined emphasis on primary care, home care, and the rapid movement of nonacute hospital patients into less expensive facilities or programs.[8]

This two-pronged assault on rising hospital costs appears to attack the key causes of hospital cost inflation as identified by most cost containment analysts, and as such it should show signs of working as individual segments are put in place. By simultaneously controlling the hospital's internal operating costs and moving substantial numbers of patients into less expensive facilities and programs, it should be possible to slow the hospital system's consumption of the nation's health care resources.

Unfortunately, there are strong indications that this dual approach has not achieved its goals.[9] Indeed, although programs thus far have been implemented only piecemeal, results from a number of studies suggest that regulatory efforts to reduce either the rate of hospital cost increases or the hospital system's share of national health expenditures have at best been marginally successful.

From a rate-setting perspective, for instance, Dowling (1979) cites performance evaluations of the prospective reimbursement system in downstate New York showing that the annual rate of hospital cost increase did slow, but only slightly, from 15 percent to 13 percent. Dowling concludes that even under the best of conditions the results from such programs will likely be only a 5 percent drop in the rate of increase, from 15 percent to 10 percent per year. Biles, Schramm, and Atkinson (1980), by contrast, evaluated the experience of states with and without hospital rate-setting programs and arrived at a similar conclusion. Specifically, rate-setting states had an overall cost increase of 11.2 percent per year, compared with 14.3 percent per year for other states. Ruchlin and Rosen (1980) concluded that their own results in a study of hospitals in New York state "seem to confirm those cited in other studies that question the effectiveness of state cost containment programs implemented through the reimbursement process" (52). Hellinger (1979) concluded similarly that prospective rate-setting systems are capable of ultimately reducing the rate of hospital cost inflation by no more than 2-4 percent per year. Bauer (1977) pointed to numerous instances in which prospective programs have had little positive effect upon cost inflation and have occasionally had a negative effect. Finally, Sloan (1983) found that "successful" rate-setting programs achieved all their savings by reducing per diem or per admission payment *rates,* but they did not curb growth in either admissions or length of stay.

While a reduction of two to three percentage points from a 15 percent annual rate of increase may yield significant dollar savings — at least in the short run — it is highly doubtful that the associated savings will be sufficient to resolve the political crisis that surrounds public funding for health care. As table 1 indicates, health care costs continue to increase at twice the general inflation rate, and the percentage of national income devoted to health continues to grow almost unabated. Without entering into the debate over How much is enough? it seems fair to conclude that existing rates of expenditure reduction are unlikely to forestall further controls over federal and state health care programs.

Thus, rate setting alone is not the answer. Contrasted with a rate-setting perspective is direct intervention. Here Salkever and Bice (1978), for example, concluded that certificate of need programs (one form of direct intervention) do not reduce the hospital system's overall rate of capital investment but simply deflect such investment from new beds into other capital facilities, which, as Hughes et al. (1978) noted, actually raises the hospital's overall operating cost per patient-day.

Hughes et al. (1978) also found that utilization review (another form of direct intervention) as conducted by individual hospitals had only a minimal effect on overall costs. Moreover, an Institute of Medicine (1976) study, McGarrah et al. (1976), and a Congressional Budget Office (1981) study also found that PSROs have been equally ineffective as cost containment measures. Similarly, other forms of direct intervention have had limited success. In short, regulation as practiced to date in the United States leaves much to be desired. To understand why this is so, we must look to the hospital sector and its response to regulatory efforts.

As might be expected, the two-pronged regulatory attack on the hospital's overall revenue has evoked a strong response. Far from passively assenting to limitations upon their overall growth and cash flow, many hospitals have sought to turn both provider competition and regulatory control programs to their own advantage. One good indicator of the magnitude of this response has been the accelerated development of marketing strategies for hospitals. Goldsmith (1980), for example, suggests that hospitals should adopt a marketing strategy for their services like that of the private sector. He advises hospitals to react to provider competition and cost containment programs much as a private corporation does when it is faced with an equivalently maturing market: the hospital should diversify its operations by absorbing institutions that have related operations or operate in related markets, and it should expand vertically into manpower and other supply operations (nursing and medical schools, for example). Goldsmith also suggests such patient-generating activities as running health-screening programs for schools and employers, operating transportation services such as vans and helicopters equipped for intensive care, providing financial assistance to medical residents who agree to set up a practice within the hospital's service area, and establishing freestanding emergency rooms and outpatient clinics to compete with other available primary care facilities.

Beyond the development of new revenue-generating programs, many hospitals have also sought to maximize their reimbursement payments under existing rate regulation programs. Ruchlin and Rosen (1980) conclude that in New York the required uniform statistical reports and uniform financial reports are "completed with a definite objective in mind—reimbursement maximization" (44), and hospital consulting firms routinely use computer programs that help individual hospitals increase their reimbursement revenues. The most recent example of this approach is the phenomenon known as "DRG creep" (Simborg 1981). More important, in what may be only the visible tip of an accounting iceberg, hospitals have both challenged their individual rate schedules and brought legal suits to change the way such schedules are determined.[10]

Corroborative evidence of a different kind can be found in Davis (1973). As if to confirm the suspicion that regulatory policy remains focused on the immediate effects of a more deeply rooted problem, Davis concluded that hospital costs had already been rising before the onset of Medicare and Medicaid and that the types of cost increases after 1965 were similar to those experienced earlier, only larger. This finding suggests that the forces driving up hospital costs have long been embedded within the hospital's institutional structure and that the recent injection of new funds and additional patient demand has not created hospital cost inflation but instead exacerbated an existing condition.

At the root of many of these efforts to resist the intent of regulation is the medical community. Taylor and Paranjpe (1984), in their survey of physician attitudes toward cost containment, for example, report that although physicians believe that utilization reviews are somewhat effective, 44 percent do not consider them acceptable. Fixed fees based on DRGs are also unacceptable to most physicians, as are HMOs and preferred provider plans. The greatest negative response was to government price controls, which 85 percent of the physicians surveyed found unacceptable. Similarly, Sloan's (1983) finding that rate setting had an inhibiting effect on expense per unit of output but not on volume of output can be tied directly to the cost-generating activities of the attending physician. As Platt (1984) phrased it, "The current fee-for-service system not only rewards physicians for doing more but provides extraordinary support for procedural activities. . . . The fee-for-service system reinforces the clinical bias of most physicians that more care is better than less."[11]

This idea, that physicians operate in a different financial world from the hospitals where they see their patients, has become more important with Medicare's imposition of a DRG reimbursement system. Before that time, physicians' motivations under a fee for service system coincided reasonably well with the incentives of their hospitals: for both, more care in the form of longer stays and increased use of ancillary services was, with few exceptions, financially beneficial. With the DRG-based per admission form of reimbursement, the interests diverge: what is in the best financial interest of the hospital for its Medicare patients (short stays and few ancillaries, for example) now runs directly contrary to the financial interests of most attending physicians. How this conflict will be resolved and what its implications are for patient care are questions that remain to be answered.[12]

In sum, then, the evidence available to date indicates that the two-pronged regulatory policy described above has not been able to successfully contain hospital costs, largely owing to the resistance of hospitals, with support from their medical staffs, to any reduction in their revenues. Further, the evidence suggests that an effective regulatory program must be able to account for — and to counteract — a more deep-seated reluctance of hospitals and physicians to accept limits on the growth of their activities.

A Misconception of the Market

Despite their differences in focus, both cost sharing and regulation suffer from a central misconception about the structure of inpatient medical care and from a mistaken perception that the health care delivery system performs according to some standard industrial model. In terms of regulatory efforts, most of the cost containment programs discussed in the previous section have presumed that the best way to reduce the cost of inpatient medical care — since it is delivered inside the walls of a hospital — is to place financial pressure on the hospital itself. In so doing, regulators act as if the decision-making processes inside a hospital were similar to the hierarchical pattern found within most other large organizations. Thus federal and state reimbursement regulations typically seek to squeeze the hospital's overall revenues, in the expectation that hospital administrators — like top management in industrial firms — will then force their organizations to operate with lower costs.[13] By contrast, cost sharing advocates insist that if price changes, customers will reduce their demand — as in any traditional market.

In reality, the structure of the health care system does not allow for such unicausal approaches. As we will discuss in chapter 2, hospitals have a sharply bifurcated decision-making process, in which the clinical decisions that drive the institution (and most of its costs) are made by physicians, while the financial responsibility associated with providing physician-ordered services rests with hospital management. Moreover, once a patient is hospitalized, the "demand" for services is also determined almost exclusively by the attending physician's clinical decisions. Given this organizational structure, it is not surprising that neither cost sharing nor regulation, as they have been formulated in the past, has adequately addressed health care's complex and sometimes anomalous decision-making structure.

For costs to be contained without jeopardizing the system's fundamental ability to provide all patients with access to quality care, health policy must move beyond existing regulatory and proposed competitive approaches. Instead, both federal and state responses must be redesigned to accommodate the real-world complexity of the health care delivery system. As a first step, we must discard the notion that there is — or ought to be — a single "health care marketplace." Rather, we must recognize that there are four medical submarkets, composed of different "actors" within the system. There is one medical submarket between patients and physicians, a second between patients and health insurers, a third between physicians and health insurers, and a fourth between hospitals and health insurers. Individual transactions take place independently within each submarket, yet the integrated character of the overall delivery system means that the behavior within each submarket influences the behavior of the other three. While there are "prices" within each submarket, the dominance of the health care delivery system by physicians and hospitals, coupled with the potential purchasing power of health insurers, dictates that efforts to contain costs must focus principally, if not exclusively, on the third and fourth submarkets.

Furthermore, regulatory policy must be reformulated to accommodate the nonhierarchical character of inpatient medical care. In particular, policymakers need to focus on the key role physicians play in decisions on patient care and to devise clinically appropriate yet managerially effective mechanisms for reviewing and controlling physicians' cost-generating behavior. Schroeder's (1980) estimate that 80 percent of all health care expenditures result from physician orders, with an even higher percentage applicable to inpatient hospital care, suggests that a meaningful cost containment program must place substantial emphasis on physician decisions.

In brief, a successful cost containment program must incorporate an understanding of the physician's role as the driving force behind inpatient costs, the multiple medical submarkets that characterize the inpatient delivery system, and the social necessity of adequate access to quality care. Moreover, as we will discuss in part 3, such a program must concentrate in particular on the medical submarkets between physicians and insurers and between hospitals and insurers.

The Challenge to Policymakers

To summarize, neither existing regulatory programs nor proposed cost sharing options are properly framed to deal with a health care system that is in large part under the control of the physician. Because both of these cost containment strategies rely upon indirect, external, and primarily aggregate financial pressure to change the behavior of the system's key actor, neither approach is likely to achieve substantial reductions in the cost of patient care. As now formulated, therefore, both regulation and cost sharing set the political stage for new pressures toward cost cutting that may well overwhelm the system's ability to maintain medically necessary services.

Rather than adopting economically unsound and socially undesirable proposals, we need to begin from the rather different premise that health care is a social as well as an economic good. Working on this basis, we must develop more precisely targeted and refined regulatory policies that are congruent with the existing and projected *need* for care. Such policies must enable us to contain *unnecessary* costs without jeopardizing individuals' access to quality care.

As our four-market model indicates, an effective solution would not focus on the patient. Rather, it would require physicians, hospitals, and other providers to be both financially and medically responsible for their decisions. As a consequence, the requisite regulatory structure must be less aggregate in its focus than those in use at present, yet considerably more comprehensive in its scope. It must be based on a dual strategy that, first, changes institutional budgeting and reporting systems to ensure that physicians will be held responsible for the financial as well as the medical implications of their decisions and, second, establishes a reimbursement framework to ensure that all institutions comply fully with the cost containment effort. In short, public-sector regulation must establish budgeting and reporting systems that ensure effective integration of all responsible parties both at the institutional level and systemwide.

With this combined regulatory and management approach, we would have the opportunity to control health costs while maintaining existing medical services for all Americans, including the financially vulnerable sectors of our population. In our view, the challenge to policymakers is not simply to slow the growth of health care expenditures, but rather to design regulatory systems that can contain them in a medically and socially acceptable fashion. The remaining chapters are devoted to this effort.

CHAPTER 2
The Hospital Power Equilibrium: A Theoretical Framework

Proponents of increased competition and those of increased regulation share more than the fundamental misconception of the health care marketplace discussed in chapter 1. Both groups of reformers also tend to accept a similarly misconceived notion of the nature of the key "forces" within that marketplace, particularly within nonprofit, acute-care hospitals. In the cost containment arguments of regulation and competition advocates alike, one finds the pervasive presumption that a hospital, like most other modern organizations, has a hierarchical decision-making structure that can bind the entire enterprise to its will. We will argue in this chapter that, quite the contrary, the modern hospital has a highly bifurcated authority structure that splits financial control from medical control. This basic misconception about hospital organization explains why much recent cost containment literature, while increasing our knowledge about *how* hospital costs have been incurred, has been less useful in describing the underlying factors that *generate* these costs.

This chapter is predicated on the belief that effective cost containment requires a better understanding of hospitals' internal decision making. Until we understand the sources from which institutional resistance to cost containment springs, we will remain unable to explain hospitals' reactions to past policy interventions; nor, more important, will we be able to predict their responses to proposed policies. In effect, before we can formulate an effective hospital cost containment program, we need an adequate political theory of the hospital.

In this chapter, we attempt to construct such a theory. We begin with a review and evaluation of several prior conceptualizations of hospital decision-making behavior. Following this, we suggest that Crozier's (1964) notion of a "conflictive equilibrium," though not previously utilized in a hospital context, provides a promising model for a more adequate political theory of the hospital. After exploring the application of this model to the hospital's decision-making environment, we offer some observations about the model's implications for hospital cost containment.

Theories of Hospital Decision Making

There is a sizable literature on the internal structure of the hospital. Jacobs (1974) devised a useful classification scheme for this work that results in two basic models of how the hospital functions: the traditional "organism model" and the more recent "exchange model."

The organism model of hospital behavior treats the hospital as an entity in its own right, an organic whole with its own discrete goals against which its performance can be measured. This is essentially a traditional hierarchical model of hospital decision making, in which power is assumed to be lodged in fact where it is lodged formally on the organization chart — with the hospital administrators and the board of trustees. Unfortunately, however, this Weberian presumption about the hospital's decision making is not a very suitable model to describe an organization that has two or more distinct lines of authority.

Jacobs's alternative to the organism model is the exchange model. The central premise of the exchange model is that the hospital itself — the organization as such — is just a neutral forum within which individual actors pursue their personal goals. This view of the hospital is the exact opposite of the organism model: here the hospital is considered simply inert turf upon which numerous individuals seek to maximize their own separate advantage.

Jacobs's notion of the exchange model differs considerably from previous theoretical efforts to describe the relation between the hospital's personnel and its decisions. Perrow (1963) and others focused on what they termed the physician/administrator/trustee triangle. In their view, the relations among these three groups were essentially benign: all three adopted the official goals of the hospital as formally expressed in its charter, and the only disagreement among them arose over the best way to achieve these shared goals. Thus Perrow's model, while it identified three important sectors of decision-making interest within the hospital, analyzed the behavior of these sectors as though each held exactly the same goals as it would have held within the strictly hierarchical — or in Jacobs's terms, organism — model. Jacobs's exchange model, in sharp contrast, emphasizes the tenuous connections among these three decision-interested sectors and thereby places his model's focus squarely on the issue of power within the hospital.

Many, if not most, recent efforts to describe decision making within the hospital have been structured along lines similar to Jacobs's exchange model. In general these analysts have accepted as their fundamental premise the self-interestedness of the various professional groups within the hospital, disagreeing only in their assessment of which group dominates.

Etzioni (1974) provides an overview of this exchange model with his suggestions that a "realpolitik" approach might be helpful in analyzing the hospital's decision-making structure. From this perspective, the only organizational currency is power, and physicians, administrators, and trustees all seek to control the hospital's formal structure of authority. In a similar fashion, Newhouse (1970) describes hospital behavior as the product of three competing groups; but he, like Etzioni, does not discuss the mechanics of how such a fragmented organization actually arrives at a decision on any given question. Roos (1974), looking at the result of this process, characterizes the hospital as a "satisficing organization" in which the conflicting goals of key groups limit the hospital's ability to make policy decisions.

Smith (1955) and Harris (1977) confront the issue of decision-making power directly, attempting to explain hospital behavior in terms of two separate lines of authority — medical control by the physicians, financial control by the administrators — loosely coupled via compromises and political bargains. Clarkson (1972) believes that the key decision forces emanate from a conflict between administrator and trustee; Pauly and Redisch (1973) focus on the relationship between physician and trustee; and Buchanan and Lindsey (1970) assess the conflict between physician and administrator.

Whereas Etzioni, Newhouse, and Roos perceive the hospital's decision-making struggle as having three participants and Harris, Clarkson, Pauly and Redisch, and Buchanan and Lindsey focus on two, there are several analysts who perceive the hospital's power structure as the private preserve of only one group. Lee (1971), for example, assigns decision-making power within the hospital exclusively to its administrators, who exercise that authority primarily in their own financial and professional interest. Alternatively, Redisch (1978) and also Todd and Rice (1979) argue that physicians exercise exclusive authority within the hospital, arranging both medical and financial decisions to fit their own professional and financial concerns.

By moving away from the formal organism model, each of these exchange models of hospital decision making contributes to the development of a more complete political theory of the hospital. Indeed, despite their different and conflicting conclusions, the exchange models begin to introduce more directly political notions about power and authority into our conception of the hospital. In a sense they initiate for a theory of the hospital the same process Pondy (1970) suggested was necessary to the development of a general theory of resource allocation for all organizations. By relaxing the economic assumptions inherited from the classical theory of the firm and substituting a number of political notions about organizational behavior and performance, we can substantially expand the explanatory and predictive power of our analysis.

In several respects, however, the exchange models described above are themselves insufficient to their task. For one thing, they ignore a number of important decision-interested groups within the hospital (such as nurses, medical technicians, and clerical and service employees). They also lack an operational view of the actual mechanism by which decision-making power is exercised within the hospital and of the conditions under which it might be modified or restrained. Thus, beyond their lack of agreement, these models contain structural flaws that limit their further development.

One additional point should be made about previous discussions of power as they relate to the hospital. This concerns the recent effort to inject political notions about medical decision making into the national debate on health care costs.[1] In contrast to our concern here, however, these efforts focus strictly on the public political arena at the national and state levels, and they generally consider the political behavior of only one group, physicians. Thus far, as we indicated in chapter 1, there has been little effort to develop a focus that links policy decisions at the national or state level with the associated implementation problems within the hospital. Such a focus must consider both the highly interrelated concerns of multiple interest groups within the hospital and the distribution of decision-making power among these groups. Although the former is relatively static, the latter may be quite dynamic.

Gaps in the Theory

Within the modern hospital, power as a determinant of organizational decisions exists on three different but highly interrelated levels:

1. Within a given medical specialty (for example, within the surgery or radiology staff).[2]
2. Between the various medical specialties (surgeons and radiologists, for example), as well as between the hospital's admitting physicians and its house officers — residents and interns.[3]
3. Among the different occupational groups within the hospital (physicians, administrators, nurses, etc.).[4]

As we indicated in our discussion of the exchange model, most of the attention to date has focused on certain, but not all, aspects of category 3 above. Yet only if we expand our analysis of decision making to include all the hospital's occupational groups, and all three of the levels at which power struggles occur, will we be able to address both the way day-to-day decisions are taken and the way the various levels of power become integrated into the hospital's overall operating plan. In turn, with this analysis we can develop a comprehensive model of the hospital's system of authority, which will enable us to evaluate the consequences of proposed national or local policy changes on the behavior of various actors in the hospital. To do this, we must first examine the concept of power more closely.

The Theory of Power Equilibrium

The literature on organizational behavior suggests a number of ways to conceptualize the problem of power. These include dependence (Emerson 1962; Hickson et al. 1971); decision making (Bower 1970; Pettigrew 1973); psychological need (McClelland and Winter 1969); distribution of authority (Dalton, Barnes, and Zalesnick 1968); coordination (Hage 1974); and environmental setting (Butler, Hickson, and McCullough 1974). For the purpose of analyzing the role of power within the hospital, however, with its peculiar bifurcation of authority into medical and financial components, two particular approaches appear to hold the most promise.

The first is the theory of organizational coalitions set forth in Cyert and March (1963). In this model the organization is seen as "a coalition of individuals, some of them organized into subcoalitions" that has been constructed through a complex process of bargaining and "side payments." The organization as a whole maintains its operating stability by building into the compensation system—into the side payments—enough surplus resources to cushion the coalition against any dramatic changes vis-à-vis the external environment. Intraorganizational difficulties tend to appear in this analysis when, over a period of time, the organizational slack is wrung out of the system, and the coalition threatens to collapse into its original (individual) components.

This model of power and conflict within the organization is derived from interest-group theories of power developed by political scientists. As such, it suffers from the bias in those theories toward both the atomistic individual as the unit of analysis and the presumption of voluntarism in the individual's decision to join the coalition and the organization. Also, interest-group theory tends to view political organizing as taking place around specific issues or policy concerns (described here as side payments), a notion that further emphasizes the voluntary and short-lived character of coalitions. There is, in short, a presumption of easy exit built into coalition theory that does not accurately reflect the long-term institutional character of relationships within the hospital. Thus, transferring the Cyert and March model into organization-specific terms appropriate to the hospital requires some additional analysis.

The second model, which is more directly applicable to the structure of the modern hospital, assists us in making this transfer. This model is based upon the concept of a conflictive equilibrium, as employed by the French sociologist Michel Crozier in *The Bureaucratic Phenomenon* (1964). Crozier's model has become the classic description of how a power equilibrium operates within a complex organization, and as such it seems particularly well suited to a form of organization that has two separate lines of internal authority.

For Crozier, organizational behavior is explained by a complex set of interactive processes. Within the organization, occupational groups struggle to gain control over those organizational decisions that directly affect them. To accomplish this task, each group develops its own strategy to maximize its zone of authority. Generally speaking, Crozier contends, the central component of every group's strategy is an effort to maximize the sense of uncertainty among other groups within the organization that that group will perform its delegated functions as expected. By maximizing this uncertainty on the part of other groups, each group hopes to increase its own freedom of action within the organization while forcing other groups into an informal state of dependence. The most successful applications of this strategy arise when a particular group has within its organizational functions those tasks that are the central source of unpredictability within the overall production process, such that the group's performance of its function emerges as the essential factor in the survival of the organization as a whole. Thus there are two levels of uncertainty working in close confluence: the uncertainty that the group will perform its function, and the degree to which its function is the central source of unpredictability within the organization's overall production process. The successful application of the first form of uncertainty is directly dependent upon the existence of the second, for as Crozier conceptualizes it, "Power will tend to be closely related to the kind of uncertainty upon which depends the life of the organization" (1964, 164).

Crozier's model of organizational behavior, however, is not predicated solely upon a constant intraorganizational struggle for power. He recognizes that if this were the case, no organization could survive long enough to fulfill its formal function at all. Thus there is also an internal counterbalance to this continuous power struggle that routinizes these different group strategies into a functional day-by-day arrangement of organizational authority and responsibility. This system-stabilizing equilibrium, Crozier believes, emerges from the overarching need of every occupational group to cooperate so as to ensure the continued survival of the organization as a whole, since only through such cooperation can each group preserve the foundation upon which its own present privileges and future expectations are constructed. In a sense, Crozier postulates that just as employees have a learning curve that affects their productive efficiency, they also have a survival curve that forces them to subordinate their power-maximizing strategy to the necessity of maintaining sufficient production to ensure the organization's survival. Crozier suggests that there are in fact four related pressures toward a system-maintaining equilibrium within an organization: "the necessity for the members of the different groups to live together; the fact that the existence of each group's privileges depends to quite a large extent on the existence of other groups' privileges;

the general consensus among all groups about keeping certain minimum standards of efficiency; and, finally, the very stability of group relationships" (167).

We can summarize Crozier's model, then, as one in which organizational behavior is determined by a conflictive power equilibrium. This equilibrium emerges on the one hand from the attempts of each occupational group to increase its latitude within the organization by maximizing other groups' uncertainty about its own performance; on the other hand, a group never pushes its own interest to the point of threatening the organization's survival. In effect, Crozier's organizational model is one of permanent internecine conflict within the framework of a stable systematic equilibrium.

Crozier's model thus appears well suited to analyzing the power relationships within the hospital. In fact, the power structure within the hospital — what we will here call the hospital power equilibrium — appears to be an excellent example of Crozier's conflictive yet stable model of organizational behavior. When we compare the process of internal decision making within the hospital with Crozier's case study of the industrial monopoly in *The Bureaucratic Phenomenon,* there are strong parallels in the permanent group strategies that are employed, the power relationships these strategies engender, and the consequent distribution of authority within the organization as a whole. To facilitate this comparison, we will first briefly review Crozier's analysis of the industrial monopoly, after which we will consider how his analysis applies to the structure of the modern hospital.

The key to understanding Crozier's notion of the conflictive equilibrium within the industrial monopoly lies in the permanent group strategy of the maintenance workers. In Crozier's example, the maintenance workers control the most important source of unpredictability within the organization's productive process — the length of machinery downtime — and they parlay this control into a position of substantial internal power by refusing to allow any other group within the monopoly to interfere with the repair process. They carve out this zone of autonomy by making their repairs according to a set of unwritten "rule of thumb" guidelines that are known only to themselves and that effectively free them from management supervision. Two additional factors reinforce the exclusive character of the maintenance workers' technical knowledge. First, largely because of the nature of their jobs, these workers have a lifelong commitment to what they see as a dignified profession — a commitment Crozier believes is stronger than that of any other group within the monopoly. Second, the maintenance workers have an exceptionally strong sense of group solidarity, which expresses itself in the strict preservation of the group's collectively determined strategy toward the handling of all machine repairs.

Based on this analysis of the maintenance workers' strategy, Crozier concludes that the principal ordering relationship within the industrial monopoly is that of maintenance workers to management. This relationship — being the primary focus of unpredictability within the production process — governs the overall productivity of the organization and consequently reduces all other permanent group strategies and relationships to secondary importance. In sum, the character of the conflictive equilibrium within the monopoly is set by the conduct of the maintenance workers vis-à-vis management, and it is this interaction that determines the broader set of group interrelationships within the organization as a whole.

There are a number of immediate parallels between the character of the conflictive equilibrium within the industrial monopoly and the forms of organizational behavior within the modern hospital. As in the monopoly, there are a variety of separate groups, each defined by its professional function within the hospital and each with its own permanent group strategy designed to maximize its organizational authority over decisions important to that group. Moreover, there is a primary relationship between two key groups that clearly orders the conflictive equilibrium within the hospital and that relegates all other group relationships to secondary importance. Last, the key group relationship within the hospital is itself determined by numerous unpredictable elements associated with the performance of one of those two groups. We will explore these parallels in the next section.

Occupational Strategies in the Hospital

There are at least six distinct occupational groups within the hospital: physicians, administrators, nurses, medical technicians, clerical workers, and service workers.[5] Moreover, there are several further splits within the physician category, reflecting staff privileges (admitting vs. salaried house officers), professional status (board-certified vs. uncertified physicians, residents, and interns), and medical specialty (medicine vs. surgery in particular, but also between other specialty and subspecialty practices).

Each of the six major occupational groups — and a number of the medical subgroups — has a fairly well defined permanent group strategy. Some of these strategies have been noted before, usually in articles that focus on the behavior of one particular group within the hospital; but in most instances these strategies are discussed only implicitly. Therefore, before continuing with Crozier's analysis, it may be useful to review some of these occupational group efforts.

Coser (1958) presented evidence that nurses employ several alternative strategies in responding to physician orders and that their choice — their permanent group strategy, in Crozier's terms — is determined by the style of authority exercised by the physicians within their particular service. In a largely collegial situation, the nurses expand their zone of control by taking on the authority to determine the sequence in which physicians' orders are carried out. In a rigidly hierarchical and formal system (such as that of the medical ward Coser studied) the nurses react quite differently: they retreat into their official job description and refuse any task not in that description. Implicit within these observations is the perception that nurses as an occupational group — albeit by service — were able to devise a permanent strategy that maximized their control over decisions that directly affected them: the first group by extending their professional purview, the second by limiting it.

Similarly, Lee (1971) sketched out the basic strategy of the hospital administrator. In Lee's view, administrators' constant pursuit of improvement in their salary, prestige, security, power, and personal satisfaction — all key aspects of most professionals' permanent strategies — was the central motivational force that could explain the long-term growth patterns of most hospitals.

Although Coser's study focuses on nurses and Lee's on administrators, the most frequent consideration of an occupational group's permanent strategy centers on the role of the physician within the hospital. Numerous articles discuss one or another aspect of physicians' efforts to influence hospital decision making to their own professional or personal advantage.

One example is Warner (1978), who describes the central role of physicians in the decision to introduce new technology into the hospital. Although he notes a complex set of interrelationships among doctor, administrator, patient, and even medical school curriculum, he clearly identifies the professional and personal concerns of the physician as the key motivating factor in the decision to expand the hospital's technological capacity. Guest (1972) takes this argument one step further, suggesting that physicians affect the very administrative fundamentals of the hospital: accreditation, contracts with Blue Cross and Medicare/Medicaid, "even a fund-raising campaign." Finally, Havighurst (1980) notes that the local medical associations have utilized their control over "relative value studies" to impose a de facto fee reimbursement schedule upon third-party payers.

Several authors also discuss the permanent strategies of various physician subgroups within the hospital. Millman (1977), for instance, analyzes the conflict between the financial and patient care concerns of the admitting physician and the educational concerns of the staff physician. Redisch (1978) notes that not only are administrative decisions to purchase new medical technology determined by the hospital's medical staff, but any necessary trade-offs as to which machine to purchase are usually based on "the degree of power of the various physician specialty groups within the hospital."

Beyond these rather scattered perceptions of physicians' influence over specific hospital decisions, several analysts attempt to synthesize a more comprehensive model of physicians' behavior within the hospital. Essentially, these models have been efforts to place a bit more factual flesh on the standard anecdotal argument that "doctors run the hospital."

One example of this approach is Pauly and Redisch (1973), who argue that physicians control every facet of hospital activity and always exercise their authority for their own direct financial benefit. In line with the theory of the rational economic man they rely on, Pauly and Redisch analyze each aspect of physicians' hospital behavior in terms of personal income maximization. They summarize their position as follows: "The critical assumption of our model is that the physician staff members enjoy *de facto* control of hospital operations and see to it that hospitalization services are produced in such a way as to maximize their net incomes" (88).

The difficulty with this model is its sole concentration upon direct financial remuneration and its exclusion of more complex and less readily quantified incentives that also influence physicians' behavior. In particular, the model is limited by its lack of recognition of the physician's social contract with his or her patients, the complicated interplay of different professional and career concerns, and the constraining influence of other occupational groups within the hospital.

From a somewhat different perspective, there have been a variety of efforts by medical sociologists to describe the role of the physician within the hospital. While they may differ on other issues, these writers tend to emphasize the importance of social institutions, broadly defined, and the structure of medicine as a profession in particular, without looking explicitly at the hospital's decision-making process. Freidson (1970), for example, emphasizes the importance of such structural factors as control over state licensing procedures and medical school curricula, to which Krause (1977) adds a Marxian emphasis upon social class structure. Within this broad sociological framework, both Freidson and Krause do discuss the question of physicians' power in the hospital. Freidson contends that their decision-making authority is correlated with the particular physician's ability to claim a "medical emergency," whereas Krause, though recognizing the power struggles between physicians and "subservient groups," attributes the existence and outcome of these struggles largely to structural factors in the external environment. Thus, while these sociological models provide an important intellectual overview of the medical profession, they do not meet our need for a specific model of the hospital's day-to-day decision-making mechanism.[6]

Finally, there are a few models of physicians' hospital behavior that analyze the physician's basic power strategy within the hospital as a whole. Blishen (1969) takes this approach the furthest, focusing upon the constraints that the hospital's increasingly technical and professional atmosphere has placed upon physicians' traditional prerogatives. More important, Blishen's description of the hospital as an ever-changing system of power relationships fits well with Crozier's more general notions about organizational behavior.

In Blishen's model, each of the hospital's occupational groups is engaged in a permanent campaign to improve its professional position, prestige, and status. To accomplish its goals, each finds itself locked in a battle with one or more of the hospital's other occupational groups. Nurses, Blishen contends, are becoming more highly trained and seek to increase their prestige vis-à-vis physicians, while at the same time they must fight off encroachments upon their present status by medical technicians. Technicians, in turn, as a relatively new group within the hospital, seek to establish their professional legitimacy within the hospital hierarchy, primarily vis-à-vis the nurses. On a different level, administrators constantly seek to transform their merely formal authority into real control over the medical staff and thus to establish themselves as the final repository of hospital authority. And physicians—who are the focus of Blishen's study—attempt to defend their traditional control over the hospital's decision making against the incursions of these other groups. Even the recent introduction of social workers and dentists into the hospital represents a challenge to the physicians' authority, and they must also face competition from other physicians for status and prestige within their particular medical specialties. Blishen summarizes the defensive position of the physician within the hospital: "The hospital has become a seed bed of professionalization and the physician is now placed in a position where he must constantly seek to protect his status" (84).

Blishen's model takes an important step toward viewing the hospital as a unified social and political system. It perceives the hospital as a complex set of power relations, in which each occupational group struggles to increase its advantage over similar groups. Moreover, there is an implicit sense in Blishen's analysis that the existing power alignment is fluid rather than static. In short, Blishen's work provides further evidence that the hospital functions along the lines of Crozier's conflictive equilibrium.

The Power Equilibrium in the Hospital

This review of references to occupational group strategies clearly indicates the value of Crozier's approach. His model provides an analytic tool for integrating the various group strategies into a single framework that is at once descriptive, explanatory, and predictive. The central concerns of the different groups—for professional prestige, personal remuneration, job security, and so on—are all subsumed as contributory incentives under the

Table 2 Parallels between Crozier's Industrial Monopoly and the Hospital

Crozier's Model	Industrial Monopoly	Hospital
Conflictive equilibrium	Industrial monopoly power equilibrium	Hospital power equilibrium
Dominant group	Maintenance workers	Physicians
Source of power	Machinery downtime	Patient management
Permanent group strategy	Based on: technical expertise professional commitment cohesive norms of behavior	Based on: medical expertise professional commitment professional standards of behavior
Key subequilibrium	Maintenance workers/ management	Physicians/hospital administrators

model's rubric of power relationships. In effect, the various economic, sociological, and psychological imperatives that create permanent group strategies ultimately express themselves within the hospital in a political form, in each group's struggle to exert maximum control over decision making.

The comparable character of the hospital and the industrial monopoly can best be explored by returning to the strategy of the maintenance workers. Curious as it may initially seem, given the disparity in their social standing, the physicians are the maintenance workers' counterpart within the power structure of the hospital. The striking parallels between their respective roles are illustrated in table 2.

First, physicians are without question the central source of unpredictability within the hospital's production function. Physicians admit patients, diagnose them, order tests and procedures, decide on levels of care, and make the discharge decision. Through this exclusive control over patient care, they control three of the hospital's crucial variables: admissions, length of stay, and demand for ancillary services. Furthermore, as Harris (1977) and Warner (1978) point out, beyond the effect of immediate physicians' orders, there is the long-term or lagged effect upon the hospital's production base created by physicians' control over most capital costs, in particular new medical technology and new services. In terms of the survival of the hospital as an organization, the behavior of the physicians is the critical variable.

Second, the basis of the physicians' critical role, and of this exclusive authority over the major source of unpredictability within the hospital, is specialized medical knowledge. The physicians' monopoly over technical expertise effectively frees them from any supervisory efforts by hospital management — the administrators and trustees — and makes it difficult to develop norms for their performance that could lessen the unpredictability in the overall production of hospital services.

And third, physicians as a group maintain their exclusive control over the hospital's decision-making processes by maximizing the sense of uncertainty that they will perform their function as expected. They do this in a number of ways, not the least of which is the implicit threat, aimed toward administrators, that admitting physicians may decide to send their patients to another hospital. Additionally, physicians may alter their ordering patterns for particular diagnoses (Millman 1977), insist that certain procedures be performed by nurses or by hospital residents (Redisch 1978), and otherwise alter their expected performance pattern to increase their leverage over other groups within the hospital.

Beyond these major parallels with the role of maintenance workers in Crozier's industrial monopoly, several other similarities exist. Physicians have an extremely strong commitment to their profession, inculcated throughout their long medical training, and they have an equally strong sense of its dignity. Like the maintenance workers, they have possibly the strongest commitment to their occupation of any group within the organization. Moreover, physicians are tightly controlled by strong group standards of professional conduct. Finally, the bipolar relationship between physicians and administrators is the key decision-making struggle within the hospital and effectively orders all the other intergroup relationships.

In each of these respects, the physicians control power within the hospital in much the same fashion as the maintenance workers do within the industrial monopoly. Their function is the central source of unpredictability within the hospital's production process because of their monopoly over an essential body of technical information. In turn, their control over the hospital's production "choke point," combined with a strong commitment to professional mores and standards, gives them the necessary resources to maximize the uncertainty that they will perform their functions as anticipated. Thus physicians, as an occupational group within the hospital, have developed a permanent group strategy that utilizes their present power advantages to ensure and expand their prerogatives in the future.

Building on a central feature of Crozier's model, however, we must recognize that the physicians' permanent power strategy — like that of the maintenance workers — is not the only one, and every group seeks openings to increase its own intraorganizational power (usually at the expense of the physicians). It is because of this dynamic that Crozier's conflictive equilibrium has a richer analytic texture that most hospital models, for it seeks to understand not only the physicians' controlling role, not only the structural tensions between physicians and administrators, but the entire decision-making process of the hospital as a whole.

Precisely as a result of this model's dynamic and inclusive character, however, we are forced to conclude that the physicians' dominant position within the hospital power equilibrium — far from being serene and secure — is under assault from both within and without the hospital. Inside the hospital, the other occupational groups are turning to more aggressive tactics to increase their bargaining power. Harris (1977), for instance, mentions that some groups have sought to improve their relative positions by staging work slowdowns, in which they do their jobs strictly "by the book." Blishen (1969) discusses the challenge to physicians created by the increasing professionalization of in-hospital groups, and Krause (1977) notes that nurses, who may be followed by other hospital groups, have recently switched from a strategy of professionalization to one that emphasizes unionization.

Outside the hospital power equilibrium, there are at least three emerging threats to the physicians' decision-making authority. The first stems from procedural checks upon specific hospital activities imposed through certificate of need programs, preferred-provider organizations, prospective reimbursement systems, second surgical opinion programs, utilization review activities, and the like. These rather narrowly focused state and private programs can, in certain circumstances, have the combined (if largely inadvertent) effect of strengthening the administrators' political as well as financial position within the hospital power structure. Second, the confidence and security of the physicians within the hospital power equilibrium can be adversely affected by unfavorable changes in the numbers and employment patterns of other physicians within their immediate geographic area.[7] And third, the increasing tendency of hospital trustees to respond to the competitive pressures on their hospitals by taking a more active role in hospital decision making can in some instances circumscribe important aspects of physicians' authority.[8]

Despite the increasing strength of these internal and external threats to the physicians' dominant position, we must be careful not to jump to the conclusion that physicians may lose their ability to control the hospital's decision-making process. The equilibrating aspect of Crozier's model strongly suggests that the dominant group within a particular conflictive equilibrium will adjust its permanent strategy to absorb new initiatives into the existing power arrangement. In the case of the hospital power equilibrium, therefore, physicians' control over the key sources of uncertainty within the hospital's production process may well still generate sufficient resources to enable them to deflect any efforts to loosen their grip on decision making. This is not to say that physicians' authority can be maintained in every situation. However, Crozier's model leads to the strong presumption that there will be little major change in the hospital's power balance. Indeed, Kinzer (1980) concludes rather bluntly that "limited efforts to date indicate that [physicians] are inventive in their efforts to 'beat' any regulatory system that comes along."

Cost Containment and the Power Equilibrium

The central advantages of Crozier's model of organizational behavior are its inclusiveness and its flexibility. It is broad enough to incorporate numerous internal and external factors affecting hospital performance in general, yet sensitive to the particular nuances of individual hospitals. It thus seems fair to conclude that Crozier's conflictive equilibrium model can provide the basis for a satisfactory political theory of the hospital. This model also can give us an important new perspective on the causes of hospital cost inflation. By focusing our attention on the dynamics of the hospital power equilibrium, the model helps explain why present cost containment programs — particularly prospective reimbursement and other rate-setting programs — cannot slow the rate of growth of hospital costs.

Summarized in one sentence, Crozier's approach suggests that present efforts focus upon the visible symptoms of hospital inflation rather than on the more deeply rooted professional and structural forces that actually cause it. With its analytic device of the conflictive equilibrium, Crozier's model enables us to penetrate the externally perceived behavior of the hospital so that we can observe the relative decision-making responsibilities of the different groups within it. Most important, Crozier's notion of organizational behavior strongly suggests that the hospital's reaction to any particular cost containment program is dictated primarily by the effect that program may have on the interest and concerns of those groups dominating the hospital power equilibrium and by its influence upon the whole range of incentives that structure the decision-making behavior of the medical staff. Thus this approach provides both a comprehensive analysis of the power relationships that exist within the hospital and a detailed and highly flexible model of the actual mechanisms that integrate these relationships into a functioning organization.

In effect, Crozier's model provides the theoretical transition Jacobs sought. It moves us from the earlier organism model of unified decision making to an analysis of decisions in terms of their impact upon the complex constellation of separate interests and groups balanced within the hospital power equilibrium.

Once we adopt Crozier's perspective on the hospital's decision-making process and on the role of permanent group strategies within it, it becomes apparent that hospital costs cannot be successfully contained through programs of revenue control or patient cost sharing. To further complicate the current situation, prospective reimbursement programs, in particular, run the risk of becoming trapped in what Crozier terms a "bureaucratic vicious circle" (187). Working from his notion of a conflictive equilibrium and the effort by each occupational group to maximize its zone of discretion within the organization, Crozier cautions that inappropriate reliance upon a strictly Weberian set of formal rules and regulations can trigger a downward structural spiral. The impersonal rules encourage occupational groups to develop zones of discretion within or around these rules, which are then countered with a new round of standardizing regulations, and so on until the organization becomes frozen into a completely inflexible structure.

In many respects this bureaucratic vicious circle is now taking hold within present hospital cost containment efforts, as a result of attempts both by various state rate-setting agencies and by Medicare's DRG-based reimbursement methods to control aggregate hospital expenditures. To the extent that the hospital power equilibrium is calibrated by occupational group priorities other than cost containment, and to the extent that physicians maintain their control over the primary source of financial uncertainty within the hospital (tests, procedures, level of care, length of stay, etc.), there will be a natural tendency for the rate setters to seek stricter and more standardized controls over physicians' delivery of inpatient medical care. The danger, from a power equilibrium perspective, is that each attempt to tighten the financial controls on physicians will provoke a new effort to evade these controls, until concerns of quality and accessibility disappear under the pressures to rationalize physicians' cost-inducing behavior.

Indeed it seems clear that this threat is no longer hypothetical, inasmuch as the response of the hospital system to the present effort to regulate its revenues has already provoked several rounds of regulatory tightening. The DRG reimbursement scheme mentioned above, the bidding process for Medi-Cal (Medicaid) patients in California (Unger 1982), and the cap on hospital expenditures in Massachusetts (Iglehart 1982), are all examples of steps toward the all-encompassing standardization that Crozier postulates.

In light of this situation, the success of future cost containment programs may well depend upon their developing mechanisms that can effectively incorporate physicians — and more broadly, the hospital power equilibrium — into cost containment efforts without at the same time establishing a new bureaucratic monolith that will interfere with the quality of care. This may be a difficult task, since in many instances the only apparent practical solution to problems stemming from the physician's professional autonomy is to impose some type of standardized bureaucratic controls.

Although this tension between professional and bureaucratic norms has been remarked upon previously, Crozier's model gives us a unique vantage point from which to perceive and subsequently to resolve the problem. Through Crozier's lens, the best alternative to this downward bureaucratic spiral — to what might be characterized as the ultimate unintended consequence of the cost containment effort — is to transform the hospital power equilibrium itself into an instrument for cost control. On the face of it, this meliorist solution may appear unlikely: if the whole thrust of Crozier's analysis is to demonstrate the permanent and unyielding pursuit of power within the organization, how can we convince that drive for power to bow suddenly before the constraints of cost containment? The most effective argument for this approach, however, is the simple fact that it can produce the greatest change in operating results with the least change in the hospital's organizational structure. If behavior within the hospital power equilibrium could be successfully modified, the overall financial consequences of the hospital's decision making could be controlled without the need to substantially alter its basic power balance. Moreover, by minimizing the degree of structural change, such an approach would limit the potential for unintended consequences that could negatively affect the quality or accessibility of care.

We might conceptualize this effort to redirect the hospital power equilibrium as analogous to a DNA transplant. If we can understand how this equilibrium functions, we can design a schedule of incentives that, when implanted within the present hospital structure, will alter the outcome of the power process — its financial product — without substantially affecting the process itself. In short, much as a DNA transplant harnesses the cell's natural processes to a new end, this solution would harness the present hospital power structure to a more effective cost containment program.

On a more immediate basis, Crozier's model has a tremendous potential to guide the formulation and evaluation of cost containment policies. With a working knowledge of the hospital power equilibrium and of the dominant role physicians play within it, an analyst could predict much more clearly the likely political and medical as well as financial results of some new or newly modified programs. Additionally, a policy designer would be better able to structure a program to as to mitigate the potential for creating perverse incentives or generating unintended consequences. Policy designers would be able to test the intended results of a new incentive reimbursement system, for example, against the existing structure of incentives within the hospital, and would consequently be more likely to develop a program that could achieve in practice what is intended in theory.

There is a substantial theoretical gap, however, between the schematic model of the hospital power equilibrium we have just described and the requirements for a model that can directly predict the consequences of specific policies and programs. The model presented here is a generic one, what might best be described as an "ideal type." Yet if policymakers are to successfully design a cost containment program for a set of real hospitals, they must rely on a considerably more specific model, tailored closely to the particular configuration of intrainstitutional forces within different categories of United States hospitals. As a result, at least two types of additional information are needed: first, some reasonably accurate assessment of the behavioral incentives that now motivate a hospital's various occupational groups; second, a depiction of the *variation* in intrainstitutional behavior among different types of institutions (e.g., for profit/nonprofit, public/private, teaching/community, religious/secular) that define the components of the United States hospital system.

Although it is not feasible to fulfill all these tasks in this volume, the following chapter provides an initial generic assessment of occupational group incentives to complement this chapter's generic power equilibrium model. This then sets the stage for a presentation of our research findings.

CHAPTER 3
Behavioral Incentives in the Hospital Power Equilibrium

The theory of the hospital power equilibrium, as presented in chapter 2, suggests that hospital administrators are highly constrained in their cost containment abilities. The very structure of hospital decision-making authority — medical control by physicians, financial control by administrators — severely limits administration's room for fiscal maneuvering, leaving open only those points upon which it can obtain, if not clear institutional consensus, then at a minimum broad agreement from physicians.

That effective decision-making authority rests within an amorphous power relationship rather than with any specific office or individual carries major implications for the design of hospital cost containment programs. Effectively, a key to more effective programs is that they must be capable of responding to the complex decision-making patterns that characterize different hospitals' power equilibria.

When we take this line of reasoning one step further, it becomes apparent that if a cost containment program is to alter a hospital's expenditure-related decisions it must work with the major forces that determine them. If our assessment of the structure of hospital decision-making authority is correct, these forces will mirror the permanent strategies of the several occupational groups that struggle to dominate the hospital's power equilibrium. A successful cost containment program therefore must respond to the specific incentives that underlie these permanent group strategies and that motivate the behavior of the hospital's key occupational groups. Indeed, as we will argue in part 3, one critical determinant of a cost containment program's probable success may be its ability to *co-opt* hospitals' existing power equilibria into an overall cost containment effort.

In this chapter, therefore, we examine the motives inherent in the permanent group strategies of the hospital power equilibrium. In particular, by defining the key behavioral incentives of the hospital's major occupational groups, we add an important dimension to the overall theory and thus gain additional understanding of the requirements for a successful cost containment program.

The Impetus toward Institutional Growth

An impetus toward institutional growth pervades most large organizations. Lawrence and Lorsch (1967), for example, suggest that "healthy organizations are always under pressure to grow" (230). Moreover, this pressure toward expansion and development reflects substantially more than simply a passive response to extraorganizational (environmental) demands. On the contrary, the interests and desires of various groups inside the organization often coalesce into a critical component of the impetus toward growth.

One useful depiction of internal pressures toward organizational growth can be found in Galbraith's *Economics and the Public Purpose* (1973). Galbraith argues that managers develop a set of career needs that differ from the formal goals of the organizations they work for. These "technostructure needs," as he describes them, are keyed not so much to overall organizational performance as to organizational growth, because for professional advancement it is essential to demonstrate one's ability to increase the size, scope, or quality of the organization's operation. To be sure, Galbraith noted, financial performance (be it profit, surplus, return on investment, etc.) is an important element in this process, since financial viability supplies the basis (and sometimes the fiscal means) for further expansion. But financial performance — and with it organizational efficiency — remains secondary to the manager's critical goal of expanding the organization's purview.

This impetus toward overall institutional growth can be readily observed in most modern American hospitals. Much as Lawrence and Lorsch postulate, there is considerable pressure on financially sound hospitals to expand, and Galbraith's distinction between managerial and overall organizational goals — slightly modified — can in fact explain a substantial amount of this need to grow. In order to explore the source of these internal pressures, however, we must first adapt this general theory of organizational growth to the particular characteristics of the hospital. Specifically, both the parameters that define organizational growth and the designation of who is a "manager" need to be refocused to fit the hospital context.

Growth for a hospital can take several forms, frequently involving a number of related factors, such as institutional prestige and reputation, that are less important within the industrial sector. For purposes of analysis, hospital growth can be measured along six interrelated continua: the size, complexity, and comprehensiveness of the institution's services and facilities; the number, background, and reputation of the physicians on its staff; the overall quality of the patient care rendered; the extent and reputation of the research operation, if any; total patient volume; and gross revenues. Moreover, growth along these continua can be achieved by expanding or upgrading existing services and facilities as well as by adding new ones.

Different types of hospitals clearly differ in their ability to achieve growth along some or, on occasion, all of these six continua. The range extends from hospitals that for all intents and purposes are dying — one thinks of several greater New York City hospitals that were forced to cannibalize their employees' federal tax withholding payments in order to stay open[1] — to institutions such as Massachusetts General Hospital, which in 1981 signed a research contract valued at over fifty million dollars with a West German pharmaceutical firm.[2] Between these extremes lie most other institutions, which in varying degrees seek to replace equipment, expand services, and increase gross revenues.[3] As will be discussed below, however, a key issue for the design of an effective hospital cost containment program is not that one hospital grows more slowly than some others, but rather that the *desire to grow* on the six continua listed above exists in most institutions regardless of the resources available at present. In short, they all would grow if environmental constraints were reduced or eliminated.

This impetus toward growth clearly encompasses a number of different *kinds* of growth and can be assumed to reflect a great deal of socially essential as well as socially questionable development and expansion. It is, moreover, only appropriate to note that for hospitals, as for many industries, organizational stasis is not a real option, since the state of the medical arts is constantly advancing. Thus, for all but the most financially frail, the true issue is not choosing between institutional growth and stasis, but rather determining what level of institutional growth is both appropriate and feasible.

With regard to Galbraith's notion of "technostructure needs" and the importance of managers' career concerns in generating pressures for institutional growth, our concept of the hospital power equilibrium implies that a hospital has two distinct sets of managers — administrators and physicians. In fact, Galbraith's model has particular applicability to the hospital precisely because hospitals have two lines of authority. The structural tension between medical and administrative (particularly financial) responsibility can often be most readily resolved through constant institutional growth along one or more of the continua described above. By enabling both sets of managers to meet their goals, growth helps maintain sufficient institutional comity to keep the power equilibrium stable and functioning.[4] Thus, although some physicians may have less personal investment in overall institutional growth than some administrators (and attending physicians somewhat less than service chiefs), all share in the de facto linkage between the conditions necessary for their professional advancement and a reasonable rate of institutional development.

Before we can explore the implications this impetus toward institutional growth has for an effective cost containment program, however, we must first examine the range of specific incentives that motivate the decision-related behavior of various occupational groups — incentives that coalesce to become the driving force behind continued institutional growth.

Incentives for Physicians

The structure of incentives that influences physicians' behavior in the hospital is both diverse and somewhat diffuse. Many of the incentives that affect both physicians' patient management decisions (and allocation of the vast preponderance of the hospital's operating resources) [5] and their activities related to institutional policy are not so much discrete as interconnected in their influence. Also, different incentives may carry different weight for physicians from different specialties (medicine as against surgery, for instance), for physicians in private as against academic or salaried practice, and for physicians at different stages of their medical careers.[6] Thus the function of the following enumeration is not to explain definitively a particular decision by a particular physician, but rather to explore the key motives that feed into physicians' decision making on both patient care and institutional policy levels.

For convenience of discussion, the various influences on physicians' behavior can be divided into three general categories: professional, financial, and personal. Additionally, as we will consider below, the mutually reinforcing character of physicians' authority over both patient care and hospital policy decisions suggests that it is appropriate to combine our discussion of influences that may affect physician behavior in both spheres.

PROFESSIONAL INFLUENCES

Of the several professional influences on physicians' behavior within the hospital, the first and most fundamental is what has been termed the physician's social contract with the patient: the obligation to treat and cure the patient as rapidly and painlessly as the state of medical science will allow.[7] If a diagnosis is uncertain, or if a particular alternative treatment might significantly aid in the healing process, the physician, as the patient's advocate, is obligated to consider every indicated procedure and to evaluate its potential contribution regardless of cost. Moreover, the physician not only is morally obligated to so treat the patient but usually is under substantial pressure from the patient or the patient's family to provide the best care available.

Beyond this fundamental obligation to their patients, physicians are affected by several other professional factors that can have a significant impact on their ordering and decision-making patterns. A central though sometimes invisible influence upon their decisions is peer pressure to conform to the established standards of professional practice. This pressure can take a number of forms, and although it may seem negligible to most physicians in most instances, it is precisely this negligibility that demonstrates the degree to which peer-determined norms in fact suffuse the terms in which physicians think about practicing medicine.

Peer pressure is exercised within the medical profession through both formal and informal mechanisms. The formal mechanisms are in some senses the least visible, since they affect only those decisions that lie at the margins of accepted medical practice. These formal processes of peer pressure reflect the fact that in the United States the practice of medicine is regulated by physicians themselves through the various medical societies and state appointment boards.[8] Consequently, to remain board certified, individual physicians must keep their patient management decisions within established practice standards. Such formal conformity is of particular importance when one remembers that hospital privileges are often granted primarily upon the basis of one's formal medical credentials.

Considerably more important in terms of influencing physicians' specific decisions, however, are the various informal mechanisms of peer pressure. While these usually do not carry legal sanction, they often define the limits of acceptable practice far more directly than do the official practice standards.[9] One particularly strong instance of informal peer pressure is the professional prestige attached to high-technology, equipment-intensive forms of medicine. Beginning with the physician's socialization into the profession in medical school, he or she is taught by both mentors and peers to place the highest value on high-science, high-technology care.[10] Hospitals and physicians that practice "state of the art" medicine are uniformly considered the most prestigious, and as a result professional approval and advancement often demand that a physician practice high-science medicine to the exclusion of other equally effective techniques.

Another instance of informal peer pressure can be observed in the continuing controversy around alternative health delivery vehicles such as HMOs and birthing clinics. Although the nature of the challenge presented to traditional medical practice by these innovations varies, each initially generated substantial peer pressure on interested physicians not to participate. Dolan (1980), for example, notes that each physician's reliance upon his or her fellow physicians to provide medical backup and referrals has heavily influenced the decision by some not to support these nontraditional delivery vehicles. Dolan summarized the potency of this informal pressure by suggesting that "a physician cooperates with unpopular providers at his peril."[11]

The last major professional influence on physicians' decision making is their concern for professional advancement. Much as Galbraith posited, the interest of the hospital's medical staff—and particularly its chiefs of service—is tightly bound up with the further expansion of the hospital's medical facilities and services generally and of their specific services in particular. Many of the physicians' other professional and financial goals can be realized more readily within the context of a constantly growing institution: better access to state of the art medical equipment; a wider range of services to offer patients; an increasingly diverse and more interesting patient population; a stronger professional reputation for their services or departments; larger increases in fees or salaries; and other related professional benefits and advantages. In a simultaneous contribution to and confirmation of physicians' interest in institutional expansion, the appointment of an eminent physician as chief of service in a distinguished teaching hospital is regularly accompanied by the provision of new programs, expanded facilities, or additional personnel.[12]

FINANCIAL INFLUENCES

Suspended somewhere between these professional concerns and strictly financial incentives lies the issue of medical malpractice suits. During the past decade the rapid rise in the number of expensive malpractice judgments—and the commensurate increase in malpractice insurance premiums[13]—has encouraged physicians to practice "defensive medicine." To protect both physician and hospital against some future charge of having been remiss in either diagnosis or treatment, physicians have taken to ordering tests and procedures that are only marginally indicated. Although it is extremely difficult to establish reliable figures for the number of physician orders that are primarily defensive in nature, Schroeder (1980) concludes that the concern for malpractice probably has tipped the balance "from 'If it can help and can't hurt, do it' to 'If in doubt, do it, as it may prevent a future liability suit'" (33).

This same question about the efficacy of certain decisions also underlies the influence that more strictly financial incentives can have upon a physician's practice patterns. As might be expected, the role these incentives play in orienting some physicians' patient management decisions is complex. With few exceptions, physicians generally do not order tests or procedures that are not indicated, particularly if they involve some risk to the patient. However, having determined that a condition does in fact require medical treatment, some physicians may be tempted to steer these decisions in more personally remunerative directions. Since the problem is one of degree rather than kind, the specific effect of financial incentives on physicians' behavior is difficult to isolate.

Monsma (1970) supports this view, arguing that the role of financial incentives, by and large, is not to create treatment where none would have otherwise been required, but rather to channel a decision about necessary treatment into the physician's own area of expertise. With regard to elective surgery—where allegations of unnecessary treatment tend to be the greatest—Monsma suggests that most questionable operations are performed on nonvital organs in cases where the diagnosis can be subject to doubt: appendectomies, hysterectomies, and tonsillectomies being three of the most likely candidates.[14]

Support for Monsma's hypothesis can be found in Wennberg (1977) and in the popularity among third-party payers of "second opinion" programs for elective surgery. Monsma's and Wennberg's conclusions are also congruent with findings that have become known as Roemer's law—observations that in most surgical specialties, the total number of procedures is more closely correlated with the number of surgeons available than with the health status of the patient population. Additionally, the alacrity with which new procedures are on occasion adopted into general use before their medical efficacy has been conclusively demonstrated—as in freezing of gastric ulcers (Fineberg 1979) and, more currently, triple bypass surgery—also points toward a similar conclusion.[15]

Finally, Schroeder and Showstack (1978) found that, in an ambulatory setting, physicians in a fee for service group that provided its own ancillary services ordered those services more frequently than did solo practitioners and that these group-practice physicians earned a substantial fraction of their overall income from the operation of these ancillaries. Similarly, Millman (1977) suggests that in-hospital general medicine physicians, in response to their perception that third-party payers reimbursed surgical specialties at a much higher rate than general care, sometimes ordered tests that were not medically indicated in an effort to redress the financial imbalance.

Despite these shared perceptions, the arguments above suggest only a tentative relationship between physicians' patient care decisions and their personal financial benefit. Specifically, to the extent that economic benefits influence clinical decisions, they appear to do so only within the framework of the physician's more fundamental professional incentives. Nonetheless, financial concerns appear to play a sufficiently visible role to warrant their inclusion in the list of incentives that influence physicians' decisions.

PERSONAL INFLUENCES

The last category of influences on physicians' practice or hospital policy decisions consists of their personal preferences. Individual practice and ordering patterns can vary substantially, for example, according to a physician's practice style.[16] Also, according to Redisch (1978), some physicians prefer to have members of a hospital's staff perform certain procedures while others routinely do them themselves. On a more general level,

Mechanic (1980) observes that once immediate economic incentives are removed or shifted — as in a capitation arrangement — physicians may rearrange their activities to make them more personally enjoyable. They may elect, for instance, to follow a less strenuous schedule or to spend more time on intellectually stimulating or professionally rewarding pursuits. If such personal incentives reduce a physician's practice time, they can have important effects on the hospital's staffing requirements and thus indirectly upon long-term institutional growth.

This analysis of physicians' incentives is not exhaustive. It does, however, indicate the breadth and scope of the influences that bear upon a hospital physician's decisions on patient care and institutional policy. Since physicians as an occupational group exercise substantial authority over the allocation of hospital resources and also play a major role within the institution's power equilibrium, an awareness of their motivations and preferences is important. Indeed it is central to an understanding of the general issues that an effective hospital cost containment program must confront, and of the intrainstitutional impetus toward growth in particular.

Incentives for Administrators

An effective hospital cost containment effort also must be able to accommodate the behavioral incentives that motivate the institution's administrators. The structure of incentives that influences administrators' decision-making patterns is somewhat less multifaceted than that which organizes physicians' behavior in that administrators' motives are more unidimensional. The absence of direct financial and personal incentives arises both because administrators usually received a fixed annual salary (as against the fee for service arrangement of most attending physicians) and from the explicitly managerial nature of their work. Nonetheless, the incentives that influence them resemble those for physicians in that administrators also find their professional reputation and advancement to be bound up with institutional growth.

A useful typology of administrators' behavioral incentives is presented by Schultz and Rose (1973). They argue that a hospital administrator's most critical concern is to maintain institutional solvency, followed in decreasing order of importance by the quality of the hospital's medical services, its internal harmony, and institutional growth.

To be sure, few would dispute the importance of the first incentive on Schultz and Rose's list, particularly in a period of tight capital markets and increasingly stringent reimbursement controls. Additionally, concern with the quality of an institution's medical services and general institutional comity clearly bear on the decisions of most administrators.

There are several strong arguments, however, suggesting that administrators can more readily maintain a hospital's financial viability, its quality of care, and its internal harmony — and thus satisfy their own concerns for professional advancement — through the vehicle of institutional growth. For example, by improving an instituion's standing on the six continua for measuring hospital growth noted earlier, administrators can do a great deal to ensure the hospital's financial solvency. This is true in part because larger hospitals usually have more fiscal flexibility and thus tend to be more viable — as McClure (1976), Mechanic (1980), and others have noted. But growth on at least some of these continua is also essential to the survival of most smaller or more specialized institutions. Rapid advances in medical technology, for instance, often require a hospital to upgrade its services or add new programs in order to maintain the quality of its patient care and thus its patient volume (the factor Schultz and Rose posit as an administrator's second most important professional incentive). Further, the importance of growth for financial viability has been heightened by the increasingly uncertain economic environment in which hospitals must now operate. Last, growth can also play a major role in the maintenance of institutional comity. As Harris (1977) noted, the tensions created by the hospital's intrinsically conflictive system of decision making often can be reduced through growth in available facilities and resources.

Hospital administrators also are likely to find that institutional growth promotes their own professional recognition and advancement. Since one's professional reputation is closely identified with the reputation of the institution, the primary mechanism by which an administrator acquires prestige is to generate it for the hospital. Since a hospital's prestige, in turn, is closely related to its size and quality, and to the financial stability of its overall operation, the pressure to increase institutional prestige translates directly into pressure to generate institutional growth.

Moreover, service and program expansion can often ease the administrator's task in satisfying the sometimes conflicting demands of key hospital constituencies such as the board of trustees, community groups, and the medical community. For the hospital administrator, then, much as for all members of Galbraith's managerial technostructure, the key determinant of professional success is not organizational productivity or efficiency but organizational growth.[17]

One structural confirmation of the importance of institutional growth for hospital administrators is the integral linkage between many apparently routine administrative decisions and growth along one or more of the six continua. Brown and Marks (1981) suggest convincingly that even the most minute decision about capital replacement is also a decision about institutional development, principally because of the implications all capital decisions carry for staffing ratios, ancillary service volume, and other associated operating costs. Thus, even when the issue of institutional growth is not being directly considered, administrators are still making decisions that will indirectly fuel the hospital's expansion and development.

Overall, it seems clear that the incentives animating administrators' decision making are more immediately bound up in the issue of institutional growth than are those that influence physicians. In part this may be attributed to the absence of direct medical responsibility for specific patients or direct financial benefit from specific patient care decisions. It also reflects, however, the obvious managerial fact that hospital administrators' careers are more closely tied to the fates of their institutions than are those of the relatively more independent physicians on the hospital staff. For administrators, it appears that both institutional obligations and professional advancement point in essentially the same direction, and thus their behavioral incentives are all largely oriented toward institutional growth.

Finally, it is useful to note that hospital administrators' key professional incentive — professional prestige — increases their dependence on the hospitals' physicians. Since an administrator's prestige derives from the standing of the institution as a whole, and since that institutional reputation in turn derives largely from the professional prestige of its medical staff, a hospital administrator is at a substantial disadvantage within the hospital's power equilibrium. Moreover, as will be discussed shortly, the administrator's institutional-management tendency to satisfy physicians' demands for growth is buttressed by a personal concern for his or her own professional standing.

Incentives for Other Occupational Groups

There are at least four other occupational groups that participate — albeit at a substantially lower level of authority — within the hospital power equilibrium: nurses, medical technicians, clerical workers, and service workers. These groups all have particular sets of incentives that influence their behavior; however, their demands generally have only a minor effect upon the hospital's day-to-day operations. There appear to be two major exceptions to this reduced role. First, when the desires of one or more of these groups are championed by either the physicians or the administrators for their own power purposes (as when, for instance, the administrators support a set of nursing demands as a device to gain position vis-à-vis the medical staff). Second, when the behavior of one or more of these less powerful groups threatens the survival of the entire institution (as in the case of a strike).

Essentially, however, the effect of these less powerful groups' behavioral incentives upon the hospital's activities is rather small. Beyond a standard concern for a more attractive financial package, the primary distinction among the incentives that motivate these four groups is the desire of the nurses and the medical technicians for higher levels of professional recognition. Nurses in particular strongly desire some of the more prestige-oriented attributes of professionals, including greater status in the eyes of other hospital professionals, a more substantial role in work design, and greater flexibility in how they perform the job.[18] Some see the recent turn of nursing associations toward unionization as a result of the difficulty nurses have had in obtaining satisfactory professional recognition within the hospital power equilibrium.[19]

Consequences of Group Behavioral Incentives

These occupational group incentives, infused into the complex interplay of decision-making processes, have a major effect on the overall behavior of most hospitals. Far from being marginal concerns subordinated to the goals of the institution as a whole, it instead appears that these fragmented group concerns dictate the framework if not much of the substance of key hospital decisions. The evident character of continued institutional expansion as the common meeting ground for these incentives suggests that hospital growth is as much a product of intense internal pressures as of any external enticement. Indeed, this growth-inducing set of internal incentives argues strongly for the conclusion that even without the encouragement of perversely constructed reimbursement policies, hospitals would still seek to expand and develop their purview.

The impetus toward growth thus develops from a meshing of two separate sets of behavioral concerns within most hospitals. The first, in keeping with our theory that the power equilibrium is usually dominated by the medical staff, reflects the impact of physicians' interests upon institutional decisions. The second set reflects the interaction of these physicians' interests with the key influences that affect the decision-making behavior of the hospital's other occupational groups, particularly its administrators.

As suggested above, physician influence upon overall hospital decision making itself must be divided into two distinct but mutually reinforcing areas of activity—patient care and institutional policy. The first area concerns the control physicians exercise over the daily allocation of treatment resources: the number and type of laboratory tests ordered for a given diagnosis, the level of nursing care a specific condition requires, the discharge decision for a particular patient, and so on. Through their control of patient treatment decisions, physicians exercise enormous if not definitive control over a large share of most hospitals' *operating budgets*. This level of control is acknowledged in the often-stated aphorism of health analysts that "physicians, not patients, purchase hospital services." Morever, since operating budgets include personnel, particularly nursing (which itself often represents one-quarter to one-third of the entire operating budget), physicians' patient care orders can be seen as driving expenditures on both key human services and material resources. The decision to add another technician in radiology or pathology, for example, or the need to increase the nursing complement in an inpatient dialysis unit, or even the increase in overtime costs owing to scheduling operating rooms for holidays all reflect the impact of physicians' decisions upon hospitals' operating budgets. Although one might argue that the physician only makes the decision to *expend* the resource, not the decision on what that resource costs the hospital,[20] it nevertheless is the physician's order that drives the system.

The second area in which physicians exert considerable decision-making influence is overall institutional policy. At this level of deliberation, the key instrument of resource allocation is the hospital's *capital budget,* specifically expenditures for new equipment, new technologies, new buildings, and, if they require any of the prior three, new programs. Physicians' participation in policy-related decision making, as we argued in chapter 2, reflects their ability to combine their monopoly over medical expertise with sufficient uncertainty about how they will employ that expertise so as to gain a dominant position within most hospitals' power equilibria. Indeed, it is within this capital budget arena that much of the power accumulated in the patient care context is employed.

Further, it is critical to note the relationship between operating and capital budgets. In a very real sense, these budgets — which reflect patient treatment patterns and institutional policy decisions — feed each other in an interactive fashion. Capital growth clearly generates a host of associated operating budget costs: new machines require new personnel to run them; new ICUs and CCUs require additional specially trained nurses; and so on. By the same token, however, operating budgets that become overextended generate the need for additional capital expenditures. Overcrowded operating rooms, heavily used equipment, and the like all serve to buttress the argument for additional space, equipment, or renovations.

This analysis of physicians' influence on both operating and capital budgets allows us to understand the genesis of most hospitals' intense internal pressure to grow. Specifically, the process begins with a substantial number of professional and financial incentives that make physicians want essentially continuous institutional growth. Within the framework of absolute external physical or financial constraints, and with the exception of the occasional physician who may wish to keep his or her own service small and thus "safe," most physicians are under considerable personal pressure to support institutional expansion upon one or more of the six continua previously described. To be a bit reductive, the road to professional advancement, peer respect, a larger and more varied practice, and increased income appears to lead directly toward institutional growth.

Given physicians' general preference for growth, then, coupled with their central position within a hospital's resource allocation process, as typified by their ability to influence both operating and capital budgets, a key cost containment question becomes, what incentives influence the decision preferences of the other occupational groups within the hospital? Clearly, given the foregoing analysis, if physicians' predilection for growth is to be mitigated from inside the hospital, another occupational group must have at least the will if not the political resources to do so. As our discussion of the incentives that influence these other groups has indicated, however, none of them has any substantial inclination to confront the physicians' pressure for growth. On the contrary, all these occupational groups, including hospital administrators, have strong and persuasive incentives to join in with the medical staff.

As a consequence, the intense pressure toward institutional expansion can be seen as meeting the needs of each key segment within the hospital. The physicians on the medical staff need steady growth in programs, equipment, and facilities to maintain both the hospital's medical reputation and the state of the art, high-science medicine their professional reputations depend on. The administrators require growth in facilities and programs to enhance the prestige and financial stability of the hospital and thus to meet their own career goals. Concomitantly, the administrators also need this physical growth to maintain sufficient service capacity to attract and retain additional high-quality physicians, who in turn increase the hospital's patient census and thus its gross revenues.[21] Moreover, growth provides an administrator with a mechanism for blunting the more disruptive disputes over resource allocation within the hospital power equilibrium. Last, nurses, medical technicians, and ancillary workers also benefit from expansion, since it creates new professional opportunities as well as augmenting the financial base for salary increases.

Thus the logic of occupational group incentives within hospitals appears to lead inexorably to intense pressures for continued institutional growth. Indeed, as suggested above, these pressures toward development and expansion are so entrenched in the professional and personal makeup of physicians and administrators that they contribute substantially to both the framework and the substance of most hospital's organizational goals.

Implications for Cost Containment

From the perspective of this analysis, the reactions of many hospitals to previous and present regulatory efforts, discussed in chapter 1, are quite understandable. Most state and federal intervention over the past decade has concentrated upon restricting hospitals' activities along one or more of the six growth continua. Since most hospitals subjected to this regulation are nonprofit entities and hence have no direct financial incentive to expand the scope of their services, many health policy analysts have expected them to be somewhat responsive to these regulatory signals. Specifically, as external regulatory pressure incorporates measures such as certificates of need, health planning, utilization review, and prospective reimbursement, to name a few, policymakers have expected to see hospitals experiencing substantially lower rates of growth in their revenues, patient census, services, and facilities.

In fact, however, as chapter 1 indicated, this has not been the case. In almost every instance hospitals have devised mechanisms to evade or mitigate the effect of regulatory controls on their continued growth. Attempts to restrict the expansion of physical facilities through certificate of need programs, for example, have succeeded only in deflecting new growth from beds into quality-enhancing services and facilities.[22] Similarly, attempts to restrict growth in gross revenues by controlling reimbursement from major third-party payers has resulted in substantial cross-subsidization of cost-based payers by charge payers (Ginsburg and Sloan 1984). Attempts to further restrict overall revenues through charge-control mechanisms have accelerated a process of institutional restructuring, in which hospitals "unbundle" various nonmedical or profit-making operations, placing them off budget so as to remove them from the purview of government regulators.[23] Attempts to restrict growth in patient census through PSROs and utilization review programs have generated sophisticated hospital marketing strategies, replete with proposals for vertical integration, horizontal acquisitions, hospital-based capitation arrangements, patient transport services, and numerous other patient-generating activities.[24] Additionally, beyond their efforts to evade regulatory control, hospitals have continually resorted to litigation to postpone the implementation of regulatory programs they are as yet unable to evade.[25]

As this enumeration of evasive hospital maneuvers suggests, the purely technocratic approaches to hospital cost containment have not worked. Rather, a successful cost containment policy must respond to some of the behavioral issues raised here. Indeed, a behavioral approach both to hospital decision making and to an effort to comprehend the factors within hospitals that frame these decisions can have a far-reaching influence on the design of future cost containment efforts. In particular, a behavioral analysis suggests that external regulation is unlikely to succeed as long as it is based on the hierarchical presumption of a unified chain of hospital decision-making authority and on an aggregate approach to controlling both operating and capital budgets. In fact, each time new "technocratic" regulation is pursued it presents an open invitation to the forces that dominate hospital decisions to find a way around it and accelerates the danger of becoming trapped in Crozier's bureaucratic vicious circle.

This behavioral analysis in no way suggests that cost sharing and other competition-based proposals discussed in chapter 1 will provide a suitable cost containment solution. On the contrary, a market-oriented delivery system would be even less adept than present regulatory mechanisms at restraining the occupational group incentives that generate institutional growth. Thus, if cost containment is to accomplish its task and, most important, if it is to do so without severely truncating the ability of the health care delivery system as a whole to meet the necessary medical requirements of all segments of the population, then present regulatory efforts must be dramatically refocused. Instead of envisioning an abstract organizational entity called "the hospital," with goals distinct from those of its flesh and blood members, effective regulation must be reframed to accommodate the behavioral incentives of the hospital's different occupational groups. Instead of vainly seeking to gain control over the aggregates of an institution's capital or operating budget, effective regulation must recognize and counter the occupational group incentives that determine those budgets. In sum, the advantage of this behavioral analysis is that it identifies a number of key elements contributing to the explosion of hospital costs and suggests an avenue of resolution that would enable regulatory efforts to move beyond symptoms to the primary sources of the problem.

In part 2 we will look more closely at how these behavioral forces manifested themselves within two nonprofit institutions, one an urban teaching hospital, the other a suburban community hospital. In effect, before we can discuss the requisite efforts to *control* the hospital's power equilibrium, we must first examine the particular decision-making structures that exist within the most common types of hospitals in the United States.

PART 2
The Case Studies

The case studies in this part are based on a series of interviews that took place in 1981 and 1982 in two hospitals: a medium-sized (six hundred beds) urban teaching hospital and a smaller (three hundred beds) suburban community hospital. Both hospitals have been disguised; they are called, respectively, Oak Memorial Medical Center and Peninsula Community Hospital.

In each hospital we interviewed individuals at several levels, including chiefs of service, staff physicians, administrative and fiscal personnel, nursing staff, and nursing administrators. In Oak Memorial this process required thirty-five interviews; in Peninsula, twenty-seven interviews were conducted. The individuals to be interviewed received cover letters and a list of questions based on our research interests, designed to help them structure their thinking before the interview. The interviews themselves were unstructured, however. After a short introduction, we generally asked an open-ended question such as, Can you tell us how the resource allocation process works? We would then follow the interviewee's lead, pursuing the area he or she seemed to know best. In this way we were able to both capture variety and take advantage of each person's particular area of expertise or concern.

As our interviews progressed in each hospital, we would bring up items relevant for particular interviewees. If, for example, we had been told that a certain individual had helped establish a particular program, we would ask him or her to describe the program's development. Because several new program endeavors were identified at Peninsula, we were able to capture more specific information there than at Oak Memorial; this is reflected in the case studies.

The result is four "case histories." The first two, chapters 4 and 5, describe the decision-making *structure* of each institution and the kinds of interactions taking place among various occupational groups at the time of our study. The second two, chapters 6 and 7, focus on the *process* of programmatic decision making. For Oak Memorial, the description is relatively general, centering on the views of various occupational groups in the hospital and paying particular attention to the "dowries" provided to incoming chiefs of service (which in many respects were the institution's programmatic currency). For Peninsula, as we have noted, the discussion focuses on several specific program endeavors.

This part of the book concludes with a chapter comparing and contrasting the two hospitals, using as its source material the information in the case studies. In particular, chapter 8 considers the implications of the field studies for the validity of the hospital power equilibrium theory and for needed changes in both current hospital management practices and health policy at the state and national levels. These considerations introduce part 3, in which we present our conclusions and recommendations.

CHAPTER 4
The Decision-Making Structure at Peninsula Community Hospital

The Setting

Peninsula Community Hospital sat in a pleasant area at the edge of a suburban business district. It had close to three hundred beds, most in a large modern building at the center of the hospital grounds. The hospital had many of the standard medical services one expects in a general acute-care facility of its size: a sizable radiology department, an up-to-date pathology laboratory, five operating rooms, an inpatient psychiatry wing, a suite of labor rooms, and a well-equipped emergency room. Additionally, an older auxiliary building housed a number of physicians' offices.

With the exception of several small programs of short duration, Peninsula had no teaching arrangement. All its attending clinicians were compensated on a fee for service basis except two psychiatrists (out of sixteen) who had administrative responsibilities and two pulmonary specialists. Of the ancillary services, pathology and radiology were organized as independent group practices working on contract, with anesthesia the only service that was salaried directly to the hospital.

Peninsula was an "open staff" hospital with approximately one hundred physicians. The medical staff met quarterly, delegating most operational responsibility to an executive committee that met monthly. As is common in many community hospitals, chiefs of service were elected for two-year terms, and the position usually rotated within each service. Additionally, there was a rather comprehensive committee structure, which exercised authority or rendered advice over a large range of hospital-related issues. Committee memberships varied, but they tended to include physicians as well as nurses, and other ancillary personnel as appropriate. An organization chart is shown in figure 1.

Despite its considerable size, Peninsula was not the only general hospital in its area. There were acute-care institutions ten miles to each side, as well as several large teaching hospitals in the central city nearby. Additionally, the state had a rate-setting system that imposed a variety of reporting and revenue constraints on the hospital's administration. Finally, Peninsula, like many suburban hospitals in the United States, had a high percentage of Medicare, Blue Cross, and private commercially insured patients but comparatively few Medicaid patients.

Figure 1 Organization Chart, Peninsula Community Hospital

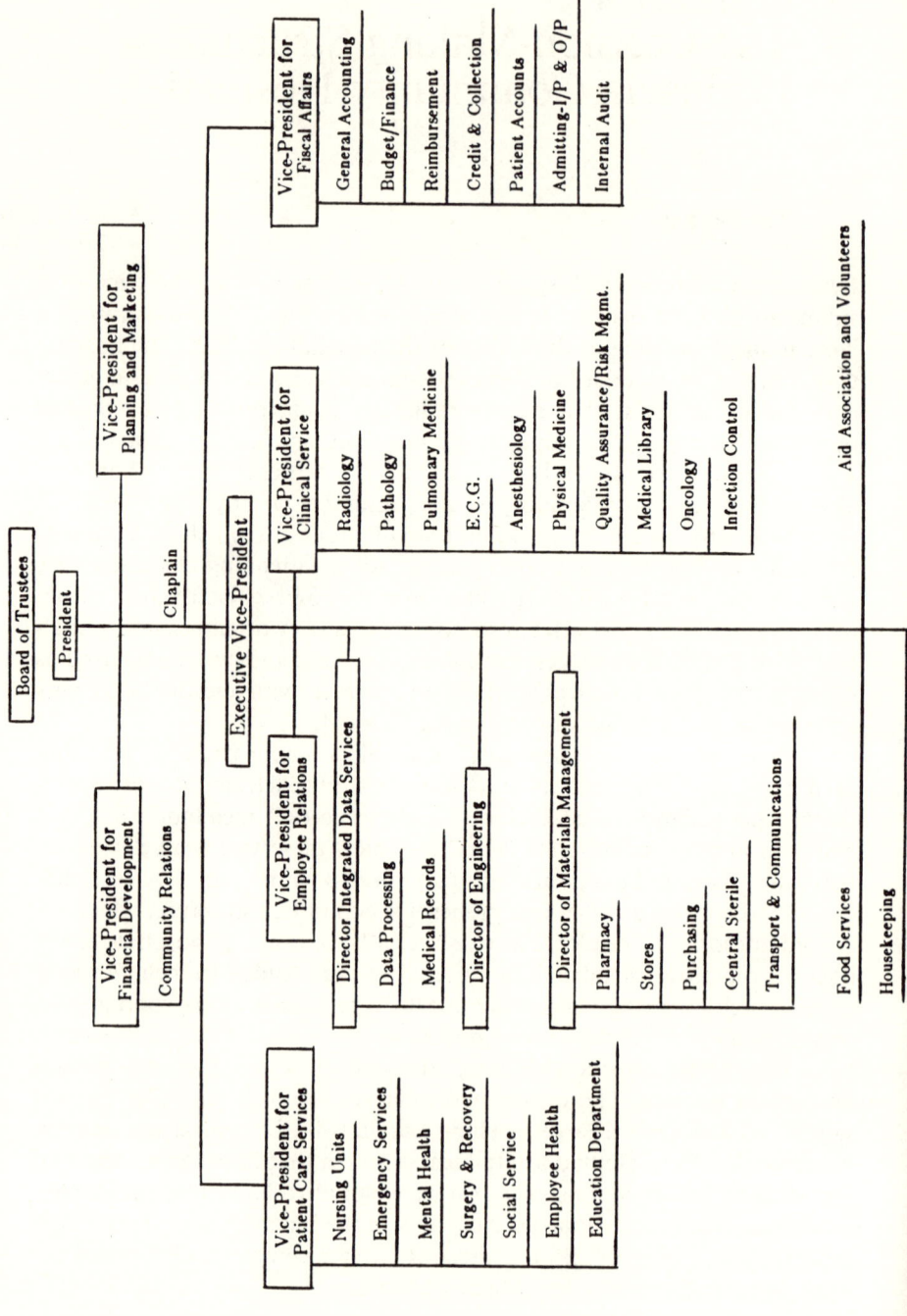

Budget Structure

The formal structure of the resource allocation process within Peninsula Community Hospital resembled that in most moderate-sized hospitals. The annual budgeting procedure began toward the middle third of the fiscal year when the administration asked all department heads to submit operating and capital priorities for the coming year. Operating results (personnel, supplies, etc.) were collated, scrutinized, and returned to department heads for further paring. In the year just past, initial departmental projections were returned by the vice-president for finance with a cover letter requesting a 5 percent reduction. Following another collating process, final decisions on all requests were made by the senior management team (president, executive vice-president, and the vice-presidents for finance, nursing, and clinical affairs).

The capital budget was dealt with more informally. Initial departmental requests were compiled by a senior member of the administrative team and filed for further reference. Once the fiscal year began each capital item was reviewed and approved ad hoc, often with a request to the department for additional justification. There was, formally speaking, no final capital budget available for general inspection.

Both within and beyond this formal budgeting process, the hospital's overall resource allocation decisions were characterized by a number of complex organizational interactions. As might be expected, Peninsula's physicians played a substantial role in these interactions; however, the format they used to pursue their goals varied considerably, according to the circumstances involved. As such, the structure and impact of physicians' behavior at Peninsula can be viewed along three dimensions: interactions between physicians and administrators, interactions within the medical staff, and interactions between medical staff and support staff.

Interactions between Physicians and Administrators

One central indicator of the physicians' decision-making role at Peninsula Community Hospital was their general level of satisfaction with their departments' facilities. In this capital-related area, most of their comments were positive: the key hospital-based ancillary departments (radiology, pathology, and anesthesia) as well as surgery all felt that their present capital situation was adequate. In the words of one hospital-based chief, "We've always gotten what we needed, within reason. There's been no major problem for capital resources. There's always a bit of trouble in terms of budgeting; for example, they may make us wait a few months until the cash flow picks up, but generally they've been pretty good at getting us what we really need." A second chief painted a similar picture: "Of course, it's a blessing that this is a pretty well-heeled hospital. The fact of the matter is that they really don't bother us. I can't think of an instance where we haven't been able to get a piece of equipment that we needed."

To be sure, none of these departments was entirely satisfied with its situation. As might be expected given their increasingly technological nature, radiology, pathology, anesthesiology, and surgery all had major capital requests under consideration.

What was particularly striking, however, was the unanimity of opinion among physicians in these four departments about two key aspects of the approval process at Peninsula. First, most of these physicians emphasized their belief that, inasmuch as their respective departments were revenue generators for the hospital, they ought to have their capital requests more favorably reviewed. In a logical line that mirrored a number of comments, one hospital-based chief contended, "I think it's fair to note here that we are among the largest revenue-producing departments in the hospital, professionally and technically very competent, without any false modesty, and producing a very large profit for the hospital. As a result of our successes, when we say something we are listened to with respect." Another hospital-based physician, noting the potential revenue-related consequences of not maintaining the requisite technical expertise in his department, emphasized the substantial financial implications for the entire medical staff: "Of course, our argument about our financial contribution to the hospital is primarily useful with the administration and the board. It should also have some meaning to other physicians, however, since if work conditions become so intolerable that we are unable to continue to generate revenue for the hospital, and we are unable to continue to maintain our quality of service, there will be financial ramifications for everyone associated with the hospital."

The second common theme in the revenue perceptions of physicians within these four departments was their willingness to circumvent established administrative channels when necessary. Such "end run" behavior was believed appropriate both within the administration — that is, going directly to the chief administrator — and beyond, as in going over the head of the chief administrator to the board of trustees. This latter strategy, evident in the endoscopy incident detailed in chapter 6, also included seeking private funds to purchase desired equipment.

These physicians' belief in the efficacy of going directly to the chief administrator was apparent in the comment of one surgeon: "In terms of individuals taking end runs around the committee system to the chief administrator directly, they often do it because they know it conceivably could be months to get a decision through the committee system." This shortened path appeared legitimate to many physicians, since they also thought it appropriate to push committee-denied requests up to the chief administrator as necessary. As one hospital-based physician described his position: "We certainly will pursue it further if we think it's important. . . . We'll go sometimes directly to [the chief administrator], although you try to maintain your credibility, you try not to do this every time." Of course, the degree of success achieved by such end runs was not uniform: some physicians obtained the desired results and others did not. One service chief explained this as follows: "In terms of the particular issue — which is to say when the administrator will accede to this kind of immediate end run request — the people who are successful are those who are placed very high in the power structure as individuals, not in terms of their offices in the hospital." From the perspective of the chief administrator, the process was a much more objective and fair one: "This 'end run' business is sour grapes, I'm afraid. My decisions are based on two criteria: need and return to the hospital."

The willingness to go over the head of the chief administrator was even more pronounced among Peninsula's physicians. Numerous physicians, particularly but not exclusively in the three hospital-based services and surgery, expressed the belief that such actions were legitimate when in their view they were warranted. Referring to anesthesia's ongoing negotiations for a new fee for service group contract, for instance, the chief of surgery commented, "Actually, anesthesia should go lobby directly to the board meeting, ask for time, and speak directly to the issue before the administrator decides. You do this if you feel the administrator won't help you, then you go to the board to lobby first." However, both the board and most of the medical staff appeared to frown on such behavior. According to the chief administrator, "The board has, in fact, refused this action. The radiologists did it recently and lost on it. In fact, they gained the wrath of the clinicians, who talked openly of censure." To give even greater weight to their arguments, physicians often elected to seek outside or private funding for their particular pet projects. Nevertheless, the chief of pathology summarized the overall environment: "You find out as a department head that if you don't play the power game you go under."

Physicians' disagreement with administrative decisions at Peninsula had also been expressed in more direct confrontation. Beyond circumventing the chief executive's authority, physicians had in the past tended to take umbrage at what they viewed as unacceptable administrative intransigence. This response typically involved bringing substantial immediate pressure upon the chief administrator to be more forthcoming. The chief of surgery noted that the medical staff's executive committee could, should it so desire, embarrass the chief administrator in front of the board—"a technique that's been used many times before, although not with the current administration." As this surgeon described it, "In a combined meeting of the board plus the medical staff executive committee (MSEC), if the medical staff has a good relationship with the administrator the MSEC will talk to the administrator beforehand and tell him what's coming up, what's on the agenda. However, if the executive committee doesn't like him, they don't tell him what's coming up, they bring it up directly at the combined meeting without letting him know, or worse, just attack him, and that's the way to embarrass him. These are the kinds of things that can be done when the medical staff is angry at the administrator."

A considerably more focused instance of this at Peninsula had involved a situation in which the hospital-based physicians were adamantly opposed to the policies of a previous administrator. On the day they received word of a proposed policy they viewed as particularly egregious, they responded in force. As the chief of pathology described it, "There was a noon caucus of all the hospital-based physicians, and by 2 P.M. that day there was a meeting in which about fifteen doctors faced down the chief administrator with fixed bayonets. There was no way we were going to give him any information about our time off — it was our business to run the department internally; it was our own bloody business. Everyone closed ranks against him, and he never recovered."

If all else failed, there was the extreme option of withdrawing one's patients from Peninsula entirely and admitting them to a neighboring community hospital. This option was viewed by physicians in a rather curious fashion. On the one hand, it was mentioned by a number of internists and surgeons alike. Furthermore, as one might expect, it seemed more likely to be entertained by those acknowledged as the more powerful members of the medical staff, who usually had large and successful practices and — like most of the medical staff — had multiple admitting privileges. Yet on the other hand, this option was rarely if ever actually raised directly to the chief administrator, nor was it, to anyone's knowledge, in fact actually used. The muted and rather understated character of this practice-withdrawal option was well described by the chief of surgery: "That has been discussed many times, but at lunch. It has never been presented to the administrator as an overt issue. Many times someone will say, 'Let's just pull everybody out and admit to [an adjacent community hospital] because there's no way the hospital can recover lost beds if it's been budgeted at 80 percent occupancy.' That has never happened in fact, of course, because it's too self-destructive. In the long run, if the hospital has cash problems, it hurts us." The likelihood that such an extreme step could have some influence upon a chief administrator's decision making was, however, acknowledged by this chief: "I suppose it is something, however, that the administrator must think about in the back of his mind."

A similar extreme scenario was described by several of the hospital-based physicians. For these physicians, of course, a "successful practice" was dependent not upon patient referrals but rather upon the continued goodwill and support of the hospital's attending medical staff. As a result of this different structure, extreme disagreement with the administration was likely to lead not to practice withdrawal by the physicians, but rather to direct dismissal by the chief administrator. Yet here too the chief administrator faced a formidable physician capacity to resist, in this instance based on the authority of the hospital's medical staff to issue hospital credentials. The chief of pathology described this variant as follows: "If the medical staff turned against us, we'd be gone. Our position would be completely untenable without their support. On the other hand, if the administration or trustees tried to fire us for no good reason that the medical staff could see, the medical staff wouldn't credential our replacements, and as a result the administration would have got nowhere — a Russian standoff."

Taken in the overview, the medical staff at Peninsula appeared to feel that friction between physicians and administrators was a standard aspect of community hospital life to which physicians had no alternative but to respond in kind. One hospital-based physician noted that "it has always been a maxim that administration and hospital-based physicians always are in an adversary role with respect to each other." And another seemed to summarize the feelings of many members of the medical staff with the following generalization:

> Unfortunately the relationship between this department and the administration sometimes seems to reflect what are the general types, the kinds of extreme cases, that are usually seen as characterizing administrator and doctor relations. Essentially, at a very basic level, the relationship between the medical staff and the administrators is very strained. Administrators believe that anything physicians want, they wanted it yesterday, they need it immediately, and they have no tolerance for time. On the other hand, physicians believe that administrators don't do a damn thing; they just sit there, spin their wheels and can't make the basic decision. Physicians are people who make decisions every day and can't understand why administrators can't decide what needs to be done and do it. These are the extremes, yet there's a certain amount of truth to that in these relationships.

Interactions within the Medical Staff

Although the physician/administrator relationship was clearly the determinant axis of decision-making power within Peninsula Community Hospital, there were several other areas of interaction over resources. One of the most interesting, given the unanimity with which the medical staff often opposed the administrator, was within and among different medical specialties. Here the issues in dispute generally concerned physicians' practices, and in particular patient referrals.

STRUCTURAL TENSIONS

There were, first, the standard structural tensions between medicine and surgery and between the fee for service clinicians and the hospital-based physicians. The antagonism between internists and surgeons appeared in a variety of ways, muted and not so muted. One respected surgeon, for example, described the divergent modus operandi at Peninsula in the following terms: "There is a big difference between medicine and surgery. The surgeon will do a workup in twenty-four to forty-eight hours, whereas the internist will take three to four days. Internists will order only one test at a time and look at those test results before they order the next. Surgeons tend to be much more rapid about it. Maybe personality differences among the different specialties enter into this: internists tend to be more plodding and precise, whereas surgeons tend to be more rapid in their decision making."

The other side of the clinical coin at Peninsula involved the lack of respect medical clinicians felt for some of Peninsula's surgeons. In particular, a recent survey conducted by the administration had determined that many physicians in the department of medicine at Peninsula did not hold the surgical staff in particularly high esteem, and that as a result they tended to refer patients needing surgery elsewhere. This trepidation also could have reflected the fact that some surgeons at Peninsula, having smaller surgical practices than they might like, on occasion also practiced some general medicine — and thus presented a threat to the internists' control over their patients.

The tendency of hospital-based and fee for service physicians not to see eye to eye also was evident at Peninsula. In the words of one pathologist, "There are adversarial relationships also between clinicians and hospital-based physicians. The clinicians feel that we have the status and prestige that goes with being physicians, yet we have none of the problems they have of running an office, meeting expenses, or even the problem of dealing with patients." These tensions emerged over such specific issues as the proposed pathology laboratory expansion, as this same pathologist pointed out in describing the encounters he occasionally had with clinicians: "Of course, when I bump into someone in the hall, they will say to me, 'do you really need this' and look at me with a questioning look in their eye."

PATIENT REFERRALS

A more fundamental rift within the medical staff, however, was that of patient referral patterns. This issue arose both within and across specific departments and, being directly practice related, hit rather close to home. There were several powerful group practices in surgery and internal medicine that had considerable influence not only on the hospital's census, but on the referral alignments of individual physicians. Moreover, as part of their effort to increase the number of referrals, various group practices had expanded to include common subspecialties as well.

The rivalry for patients between internal-medicine group practices, for example, was intense within Peninsula's department of medicine. The strength of these intraservice pressures was well illustrated by the experience of a newer subspecialist at Peninsula who was trying to build a practice: "It's extremely important what group you're identified with. I was approached by one group for weekend coverage, and by doing that created some friction. . . . I tried to just play the fence for about four months; I tried to assess the situation, but the pressure got too great to join. Unfortunately, by joining [this group], I lost association with another group here at the hospital. I used to do some consultations with [this other group], but as soon as I went with [the first group], I lost these consults." As this physician summarized his situation, "I get pushed into a nook not due to competence, but due to the power structure."

An additional element in this struggle over referrals was the question of "stealing patients." At least one general practitioner at Peninsula felt that on occasion an internist or pulmonary specialist had, as he put it, "forgotten where the patient came from." This problem was directly acknowledged by the same internist just quoted. He noted that it was "cleaner" for him to practice his subspecialty "straight" rather than practicing internal medicine, in terms of maximizing his patient referrals. In that fashion, as he put it, "I'm not perceived as trying to take their pulmonary patients, or whatever."

In the opinion of this physician, the tendency toward practice protection can be expected to increase directly with the increased availability of physicians both in the area and on the Peninsula medical staff. As he saw it, "As soon as you add too many physicians to the hospital staff, competition heats up and everyone gets protective . . . essentially, it comes about in an overly doctored area."

Interactions between Medical Staff and Support Staff

Physicians' interactions with nonphysicians at Peninsula appeared to reflect a classic "we/they" dichotomy. The physicians tended to consider support personnel—even professional staff such as nurses and social workers—to be less than equal in any of the various hospital decision-making processes that required multiple participation. One prominent internist, for example, referred disparagingly to a major committee, which included representatives from nursing, social work, and physical therapy (among other professionals), as little more than a powerless discussion group, quite unlike the medical staff executive committee. While the format of various interactions differed considerably, the central force that drove the physicians' response appeared to be their perception of interference with their practice autonomy.

Perhaps the most complex and interesting example of this occurred in physicians' interactions with the hospital's pathology department. Here of course there could be no issue of potential practice competition: the question concerned solely the ability of technicians to meet the physician's order for a certain test. When a clinician had to be approached about a problem with an order, however, it was deemed best for contact to be made not by the technician actually performing the test, but by a pathologist. This method was particularly essential if a test sample was badly drawn or the test appeared unnecessary.

The underlying issue, in the view of one pathologist, was that "for some reason, clinical physicians don't mind negotiating or compromising with another physician; however, it presents a major psychological problem for most physicians to compromise or even discuss issues with someone who is not a physician."

Since attending physicians were not receptive to communications from the laboratory technicians, the pathologists had to assume the role of intermediary. This same pathologist continued: "One of my roles is to bridge the gap between physicians and technicians in the lab. I encourage the lab techs to come to me, and to call me on nights and weekends, if there is a problem that they can't resolve with a clinical doctor—if a sample is improperly drawn, or if a test appeared to be unnecessary. It's interesting that physicians will deal with us very rationally, and yet at times they will not deal with the technicians rationally at all. . . . If I can offer the doctor a legitimate less costly option, in terms of testing, I'll call him up, and 90 percent or 100 percent of the time he'll agree with another physician."

In this instance the issue for clinical physicians appeared to involve not only the willingness to allow someone from pathology to act as a consultant, but also an insistence that this consultant be another physician. The attending physicians were not willing to discuss a clinical decision with a nonphysician professional. A similar pattern existed in the radiology department.

A related set of issues revolved around physicians' willingness to discuss particular patient questions with nurses. In a number of instances, members of the nursing staff described situations in which they were unable to approach clinicians about a problem or patient. On several occasions nurses stated that "they knew" which physicians would be receptive, and in at least two instances the figure mentioned was 30 to 40 percent of the medical staff. They also noted that it was strictly personality that determined which physicians nurses would successfully approach.

Nurses at Peninsula felt considerable animosity toward physicians, in some measure owing to these issues. Some nurses mentioned, for example, that certain physicians tended to order nurses about in a demeaning fashion. Several also expressed a belief that the fee for service mode exacerbated this problem, since physicians were their "own bosses," responsible only to themselves and not to the hospital. Although Peninsula's senior nursing administrator observed that in her opinion "a lot of the nurses' complaints on other issues in the hospital reflected the salary issue" and said that the nursing and medical staffs at Peninsula "basically like each other," she nonetheless felt compelled to add, "I think the physicians do treat the nurses somewhat inappropriately."

Physicians were considerably more emphatic in their response to any potential competition for patients from other hospital-based professional groups. In the instances of proposals for an outpatient mental health clinic and for birthing cottages — as detailed in chapter 6 — clinicians were adamant about the perceived threat to their practices by hospital-based psychologists and by midwives. Another instance included such social services activities as discharge planning, child-abuse intervention, and social service's desire to offer outpatient counseling (again opposed by private psychiatrists). In each situation physicians reacted strongly to what they perceived as intrusion of a health-related professional group into patient care decisions. Surveying the generalized nature of these responses, one hospital-based physician (who as yet was unaffected by such competition) concluded: "There is an evolution going on now, and physicians are having a difficult time dealing with it. There are a lot of areas that are now seen as encroachments on the physician's professional status — outpatient clinics, mental health services, industrial services, nursing, all this has created an unpleasant situation for some physicians."

Medical Staff Cost Containment Issues

The question of cost containment, while not in any sense a dominant concern for Peninsula's physicians, did play a role in their overall perception of present-day practice. The range of physicians' concerns extended from relatively minor issues — for example, the timely discharge of a Medicare patient — to broader worries about potential long-term threats to the hospital's service capabilities and ultimately to the institution's survival. Here again, however, in cost containment matters as elsewhere, the question became a burning issue only when it contained a perceived threat to the physicians' practices. Two instances of physicians' interaction with cost containment issues at Peninsula illustrate this point vividly: the utilization review program and capital budget matters.

UTILIZATION REVIEW

Peninsula's utilization review (UR) program was no longer connected with the rapidly dying professional standards review organization (PSRO) system that had spawned it. Instead, the primary impetus to retaining UR was a Joint Commission on the Accreditation of Hospitals (JCAH) responsibility regarding quality assurance and the hospital administration's growing concern with Peninsula's extremely high length of stay (LOS) figures.

The UR program itself resembled those of other similar-sized institutions. UR-assigned nurses made daily rounds to examine patient charts, listing on a worksheet patients with an LOS beyond the 50 percent figure for their diagnosis. These worksheets were then given to the chairman of the hospital's UR committee, in Peninsula's case a respected senior surgeon, who examined each listing. The UR chairman could either approve continued inpatient care (beyond 75 percent average LOS, the UR chairman had to sign a new extension for each additional week) or call the attending physician to seek justification. After discussing the case with the attending physician, if continued hospitalization appeared unjustified, the UR chairman wrote a letter to the attending physician terminating the patient's insurance reimbursement.

In the recent past, the UR program at Peninsula had not been perceived as particularly effective. Few of the worksheet questions resulted in a termination letter, and the hospital's LOS remained high. Most physicians viewed the program as unpleasant but tolerated it as a necessary evil. Their passive acceptance, however, may have reflected the infrequency with which its official restraints were invoked.

The UR chairman admitted that this program had had substantial difficulty in affecting physicians' practice patterns and that, should physicians so desire, they could readily evade UR scrutiny. As the UR chairman put it, "The guys have learned some of the key phrases that will help keep us off their backs. Some of the things that the physicians have learned to say are, for example, 'patient too old and decrepit to prepare for studies at home,' or 'unable to travel.' A third is that as long as an IV is running the patient isn't looked at by UR, even if the patient doesn't need the IV — and of course the physician determines the IV." Several members of the nursing and social services staffs agreed with the UR chairman's observation, noting that in effect some attending physicians had made nonacute patients — for example, a so-called social admission — acute, often owing to family pressure or the absence of an available Medicaid nursing-home bed.

There was, in fact, a perception among some physicians that UR at Peninsula — and indeed at other institutions in the area — was stringently enforced only when the hospital was full and consequently had a shortage of beds for new admissions. As one attending physician who also had privileges at another institution phrased it, "Peninsula doesn't have the critical bed situation that they have at [the other hospital], and thus our length of stay is longer. At [the other hospital] they're very short on beds, there are a lot more physicians at that hospital; thus there's a lot more UR pressure to get patients out." This physician's perception was reinforced by the chief of medicine at Peninsula, who described the UR program as follows: "When the hospital is not full, sometimes they close their eyes, but when the hospital is full they bug the doctors about inappropriate admissions. Then the utilization review committee pays more attention."

Some inkling of dissatisfaction with the utilization review program's effectiveness was also apparent to the UR chairman. In various comments as to how the UR program at Peninsula could acquire more clout, the chairman frequently returned to the need to penalize physicians financially for inappropriate admissions: "Frankly, I don't think we'll solve the problem until it hurts the physician financially when he has a patient in here when he shouldn't. . . . I still think that the bottom line is the dollar. It's too bad, but that's the bottom line, bucks."

Numerous attending physicians, of course, were pleased that the Peninsula administration did not interfere with their practice decisions. One physician summarized the perception rather well: "I like this hospital. There's not much interference policywise, there're no medical students, everybody runs the care as they see fit. In terms of the administration, there's a very loose, hands-off policy. This has been true for all administrators since [I came here]."

In sum, the essentially marginal impact of Peninsula's UR program on the delivery of care — and on the hospital's length of stay in particular — was not a great source of concern to the hospital's medical staff. To the extent that utilization review remained largely a pro forma rather than an active constraint on physicians' practice decisions, attending physicians tolerated it as a necessary if unpleasant evil. Moreover, the "fit" between the hospital administration's laissez-faire policy toward physicians' practice decisions and UR's less than emphatic role suggests that increased UR scrutiny had not been the highest priority for Peninsula's administration.

CAPITAL BUDGET

The capital budget was an area of direct contact between physicians and administrators at Peninsula, and not surprisingly it was also a source of tension between them. The medical staff in general, and hospital-based physicians in equipment-intensive specialties like pathology, radiology, and (to a lesser extent) anesthesia in particular, found Peninsula's capital budgeting process to be both baffling and, at the same time, unresponsive to department-effected savings.

As we noted above, the hospital had no final capital budget available for general distribution. This was a source of tremendous frustration to many service chiefs, who felt, in the words of one hospital-based chief, that "we send [our capital requests] to the administrator and they disappear. We never get back a reply from them in terms of what we had approved, of what's been spent, nothing."

The sense of exasperation was further heightened by the need to justify requested items again if, during the ensuing year, they were being considered for purchase. Another hospital-based physician complained, "We go through a great deal of work to estimate needs, to put together justifications, to put together our annual budget. . . . This then is theoretically approved, yet when we come to the middle of the fiscal year, and we've put in a request for a piece of capital equipment that was in our budget, word comes back that you have to justify it again. . . . It's as if the budget doesn't exist."

The explanation commonly accepted among physicians for this two-stage process was that each stage had a different purpose. The hospital-based physician just quoted continued, "Now they claim that the budget process is mainly to satisfy externals — for example, rate setting and third party payers — and that it doesn't have the force it used to have within the hospital."

The chief administrator believed physician dismay about this capital budgeting process was largely unwarranted. As he saw it, there had been a misconception about what a capital equipment budget was. The annual requests received from the departments were compiled into a report of a purely informational nature, which was sent to the board of trustees. Subsequent requests for particular pieces of equipment during the fiscal year had to be on that informational list before the board would approve them. In response to physicians' requests for a more formal capital equipment document, he had asked the medical staff executive committee to designate several physicians to help set priorities on equipment needs, but "they all wanted the executive committee to do it — eight or ten people — they wouldn't delegate, so nothing came of it."

Moreover, he believed that Peninsula's physicians did not recognize critical capital expenditure needs that had to be completed before other needs could be considered. Two in particular at the time of the study were a new roof on the hospital's main building ($180,000) and a new air conditioner chiller ($200,000).

He acknowledged, however, that the fact that Peninsula "didn't really have a capital budget" created an environment in which those physicians who pushed hard on their requests were more likely to have them approved. He mused, "I would be less than honest if I didn't admit that there is something to the squeaky wheel theory."

Beyond this concern with the structure and process of capital budgeting at Peninsula, hospital-based physicians expressed substantial frustration with the lack of recognition for department-generated capital savings. Several hospital-based chiefs were proud of their efforts to obtain a discount on an expensive piece of machinery or to arrange for operating supplies from a less-expensive purveyor. Yet they felt that these efforts went unacknowledged by the chief administrator and his predecessors. One chief put it as follows: "In terms of new equipment, we always do our homework. We paid $139,000 for a $250,000 piece of equipment — we had bids in from everyone, we found one particular company that wanted to get in on the ground floor, wanted to have a machine in place that they could show other departments. . . . However, *we* found this deal. And it was our efforts that did that. In return, from the hospital, you get zero for your cost-saving efforts."

Moreover, the hospital-based physicians felt it was inappropriate not to factor these savings into administrative decisions about future capital requests. This same chief continued, "There does come a time when you ask for something, and you wish that the administration would remember that on previous occasions you saved them money."

Conclusions

The character of physicians' interactions along each of the three dimensions — with administrators, with other physicians, and with the hospital's support staff — can be summarized in terms of three key aspects of Peninsula's present situation.

First, there was little question that Peninsula's physicians dominated the decision-making interactions within the hospital. Although the nature of the interactions varied with those involved, the result consistently resembled what the physicians set out to achieve.

Second, Peninsula's physicians strongly believed that their perspective on a given issue was the correct one, and they had no great tolerance for those who disagreed with them. Administrators and support staff, in the view of most physicians, ought simply to facilitate the physicians' delivery of care.

Third, present cost containment efforts such as utilization review were of little apparent value in constraining physicians' behavior. The nature of clinical decision making in general, and the relative position of utilization review within Peninsula Hospital in particular, made its influence upon patient admissions and discharges hard to detect.

CHAPTER 5
The Decision-Making Structure at Oak Memorial Medical Center

The Setting

Oak Memorial Medical Center occupied a sizable compound of new and not-so-new buildings on a busy urban thoroughfare. Although it was in a reasonably well-off section of the city, there were a number of poorer neighborhoods nearby, and the hospital had a substantial number of low-income and minority patients. Although it was a voluntary nonprofit institution, with a privately appointed board of trustees, it felt a strong sense of commitment to all the neighborhoods near it and diligently made care available to those who needed it regardless of their ability to pay.

A pastiche of modern and older but renovated facilities, Oak Memorial had some six hundred beds at the time of the study. The hospital had been in a period of rapid growth, and further construction of both new facilities and more beds was scheduled to begin the following year. Oak Memorial provided the full range of medical services usually associated with a tertiary-level urban institution. It had fully staffed programs in most medical and surgical specialties, suites of state of the art diagnostic and therapeutic equipment, dozens of specialty clinics ranging from the mundane (dental) to the esoteric (sleep disorders), numerous operating rooms, and a well-regarded and very busy emergency room.

Oak Memorial also was a highly respected teaching hospital with a number of coveted internship and residency programs. The hospital was one of several area institutions affiliated with a major medical school nearby, and all members of Oak Memorial's medical staff had courtesy appointments there. More important, a considerable number of the hospital's more senior physicians were on the faculty at the medical school, and many of the chiefs of service held endowed chairs. Most of the medical staff members were full time, salaried by the hospital or the medical school or both; however, some specialty surgeons were salaried part time, and approximately two-thirds of the physicians in the department of medicine were fee for service.

Oak Memorial was in a state that had an active hospital rate-setting function. As a result, its overall budget was subject to prospective review, and per diem rates were established by the state. It also had a fairly high proportion of Medicaid and Medicare patients, and some of its services had a considerable problem with bad debts and free care.

Oak Memorial also faced substantial competition both within the city itself — where there were other tertiary-level institutions — and from various suburban institutions. Although the hospital felt reasonably secure about its patient base and its referral structure — and though it had been consistently "over census" and continued to add new facilities and programs — there was palpable concern among both senior administrators and senior physicians about the hospital's future prospects.

Budget Structure

The operating budget at Oak Memorial Medical Center was perceived by senior administrators as being shaped primarily by the hospital's strategic direction. It was initially sketched out at a management retreat in late winter, well before the beginning of the fiscal year on 1 July. At this retreat the director of fiscal affairs put forward a variety of possible scenarios for the coming year, and the group sifted through such issues as pay policy and program additions. In this fashion management determined the essential constraints under which the budget was to be formulated (for example, "This is a break-even year with no program additions") before the submission of formal budget requests from the hospital's departments.

Individual departmental budgets then percolated through the several levels of administration (see fig. 2 for an organization chart) from the five assistant administrators to the two associate administrators and finally to the executive vice-president and president. At each level winnowing and compromise occurred, so that by early spring there was a final document that satisfied the initial criteria.

The capital equipment budget was formulated separately from both the operating budget and the major capital projects budget. Essentially, the process was similar to that for the operating budget. An initial amount was determined by senior management — in recent years it had been in the neighborhood of two million dollars. Funds to meet previous commitments — for example to a new service chief — were deducted, and then departmentally generated requests were evaluated, revised, and winnowed until an acceptable list of priorities had been agreed upon for the remaining funds. Once the budget was established, accepted requests generally were funded early in the fiscal year.

Interactions between Physicians and Administrators

The basis upon which the medical staff and the administration at Oak Memorial interacted was influenced by two central aspects of the hospital's internal organization. First, like many large medical school–affiliated institutions, Oak Memorial had a tripartite mission, with equal emphasis placed in the clinical, research, and teaching functions of its physicians. Second, again like such institutions, Oak Memorial's medical staff was clearly dominated by its clinical chiefs of service. Indeed, most ad-

Figure 2 Organization Chart, Oak Memorial Medical Center

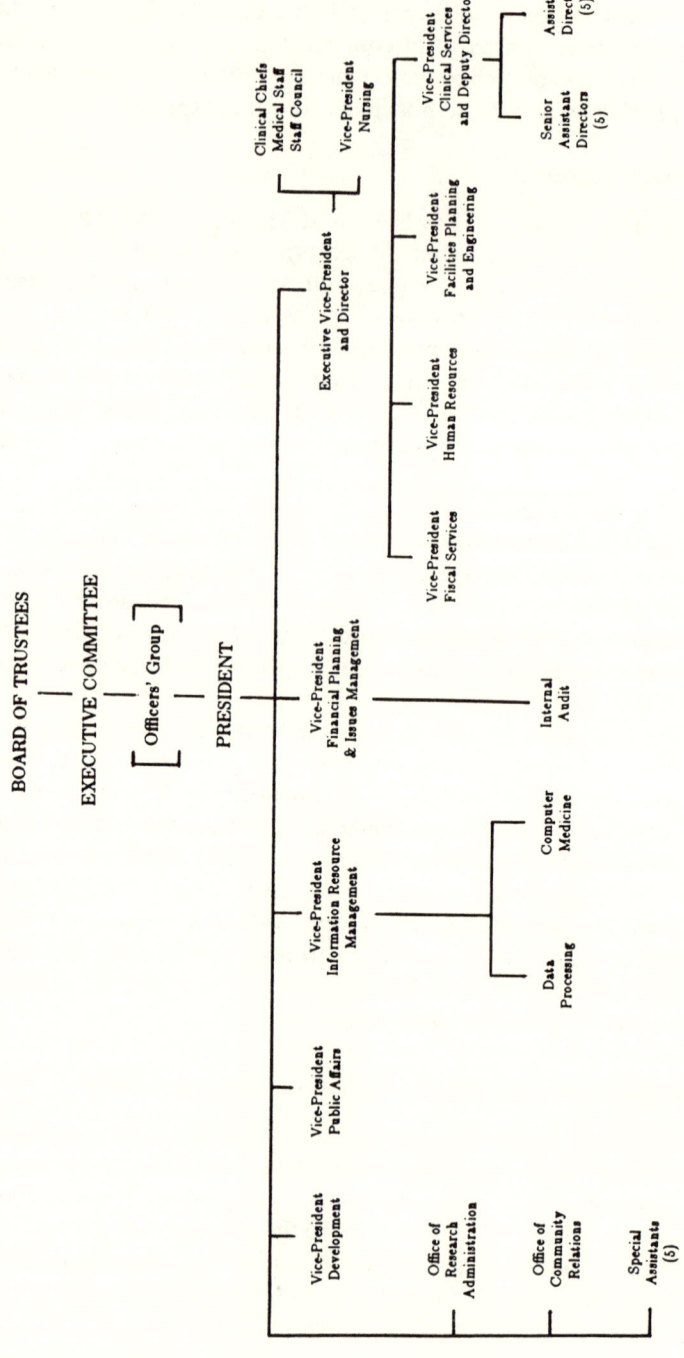

ministrative decisions of consequence for each clinical service were made almost exclusively by its chief. These two structural characteristics created a general decision-making environment in which the institution's three related but separated functions were reconciled and balanced and in which all major decisions influencing resources were taken at the level of the chiefs in conjunction with the administration.

At the time of the study there appeared to be a complex and occasionally contradictory set of decision-making incentives at work within Oak Memorial. Although the two dominant concerns — prestige and finances — were in many respects shared by both the chiefs (as a proxy for the medical staff) and the administrators, the actual meaning and configuration of each concern differed both between the two groups and within each group.

PRESTIGE INCENTIVES

The first incentive was a very strong, indeed predominant, concern with generating and maintaining prestige. Both at the level of clinical service and institutionwide, and with regard to all three components of the hospital's mission, a fundamental decision-making criterion appeared to be to foster external recognition and reputation — the operating definition of prestige at Oak Memorial. This emphasis on prestige by and large translated into servicewide and institutionwide strategies to create the highest-quality programs in teaching, research, and clinical care, with "quality" defined according to the dominant conceptual framework of the physicians' professional peers.

More specifically, for physicians in general and chiefs of service in particular, prestige was associated with state of the art medicine in a specialty or subspecialty. It was assessed by such criteria as the number of research papers published, the ability to place one's residents at other prestigious institutions after training, and the scope and diversity of patients at specialized clinics. Additionally, there appeared to be a clear sense among all chiefs except one that service growth — in terms of both dollars and dedicated space — was itself a prerequisite for a prestigious program. One surgical subchief described this interest quite directly: "Every chief who comes to the hospital wants to expand." And in an oblique but clear confirmation of this pattern, the hospital's new chief of medicine noted of his subchiefs, "They have what they need, but they constantly come to me for more, and they're constantly justified because there's always more that is necessary."

Speaking somewhat more cryptically, another chief commented that "university hospitals, if people say they are a success, tend to be a success."

Asked what "success" consisted of, this chief responded, "The trustees think it's prestige."

Perhaps the most telling evidence about the importance of prestige for physicians at Oak Memorial was that it was perceived to be the dominant decision-related incentive both by those who benefited and by those who lost out as a result. The chief of service of a small but rapidly growing department, who himself clearly benefited from the prestige orientation of the institution, characterized power within the hospital's decision-making process as the product of prestige-enhancing behavior: "Anything one does that is outstanding gains one leverage."

On the other side of the coin, one of the hospital's part-time physicians who also had a private fee for service practice, and who just as clearly felt that the institution's prestige orientation had weakened his own position within it, also characterized power within Oak Memorial as tied to prestige: "The idea is that the greater the radius between the physician and the patient, the more the prestige, but that shouldn't be. Power is associated with promotion, with money for grants, and with good jobs afterward for your residents."

FINANCIAL INCENTIVES

The second fundamental decision-making incentive at Oak Memorial, much as one might expect of a large urban institution facing an active state rate-setting agency, was a growing concern with costs and revenues. This concern was essentially ancillary in nature, however, in that it was perceived primarily as the need to provide sufficient funding for the hospital's already-determined teaching, research, and clinical programs. The financial incentive at Oak Memorial, in short, focused on the ongoing funding of the institution's commitment to a set of prestige-enhancing activities. In this sense financial concerns were secondary to prestige concerns within the hospital's decision-making process.

As the description above suggests, physicians and chiefs were concerned about their own professional activities rather than finances per se. In large part this was true because all chiefs and most other physicians were fully salaried by the hospital or its associated medical school or both (although there were increasing efforts by the administration to tie salary to patient volume for clinic-employed physicians). As a result, financial concerns for physicians generally translated into support for growth in space, equipment, programs, and personnel. This is not to suggest that concern was not expressed by most chiefs about the hospital's overall financial situation, but rather to indicate that such concerns usually did not interfere with each chief's assessment of his [1] own department's needs.

PRACTICE FUNDS

Bridging — or partially bridging — the prestige-finance disparity at Oak Memorial was the proliferation of "practice funds," which most clinical services generated by various types of private billing. (Surgery charged for the chief resident's operating time, for example, when he operated on a patient and engaged in what was essentially a private physician-patient relationship.) These practice funds were often sizable — some service chiefs had $100,000 or more per year to support various professional activities — and were considered a critical component of a chief's financial flexibility. In fact, the two service chiefs who did not have such funds (pathology and anesthesiology) were, at the time of the study, actively pursuing strategies to establish them.

The chief of pathology described his practice fund strategy as follows: "The thing I've got my eye on is outpatient tests, which in this hospital aren't sent to this lab. One key reason is that in-house lab charges are much higher than those outside — sometimes four or five times higher for certain tests. The reason is that lab costs are set high by the hospital administration to cover other losses. We're looking toward a dual pricing structure, or changing our rates."

These funds most commonly were used to support new research that had not as yet attracted sufficient grant money or personnel that the hospital would not or could not support. The chief of radiology, for example, used his practice fund to "buy out" one day per week for his clinical staff so that they could conduct research. The chief of orthopedic surgery, sensitive about "the differential for academic orthopedics versus those who are in private practice," relied on his practice fund as an income supplement and "to support people in terms of getting people funded — perhaps providing additional administrative personnel for the clinical labs, providing for travel for educational activities. One major thing that this money does is to get research started: none of the NIH grants fully support a researcher."

Speaking somewhat more candidly, another chief explained that practice funds could support new faculty members until the hospital could be convinced to pick up a salary: "I want to hire, but I have not always had the funds. I thought it wouldn't be appropriate during a time of fiscal stringency to ask for them. The department is now negotiating for several new faculty without a budget. The ploy is, if the program develops well and proves its merit, to try to pick up institutional funding later on. The position would initially be paid for by the group-practice kitty rebated to the department."

Thus the need to marshal revenue to support professional activities had led chiefs to become much more directly entrepreneurial and to develop their own private sources of funds to support their services' continued development.

Interactions within the Administration

For Oak Memorial's administrators, the relation between prestige and revenue was substantially less complementary than for its chiefs of service. Although the concern with sustaining and augmenting institutional prestige remained the dominant factor influencing decisions for the hospital's senior administrators, this primary orientation was increasingly being subjected to sharp modification owing to fiscal considerations. At the time of the study, however, financial issues still appeared to be dominated by prestige issues in terms of influence on administrative decisions. If a project or activity would enhance the hospital's prestige in one or more areas of its mission, it would still be undertaken, by and large regardless of the (at least short-run) financial impact. Moreover, to reduce its need to consider the financial implications of its prestige-enhancing activities, Oak Memorial's administration was pursuing the possibility of corporate restructuring; this would enable the hospital to establish for-profit sister corporations whose income would be off budget for reimbursement and other regulatory purposes.

THE ASSISTANT DIRECTORS' PERSPECTIVE

As might be expected, the tension concerning the proper balance between prestige-oriented and financial imperatives manifested itself differently within the hospital's administrative structure. Essentially, the assistant directors (or the lower echelon of administration) who had line responsibility for working on budgetary matters with the hospital's clinical and support departments, along with the staff in fiscal affairs, who had direct responsibility for the hospital's accounting and budget monitoring functions, were most closely involved with the balance between the two.

In large part the dispute centered on the *criteria* by which new projects and activities were to be evaluated and ultimately approved. The assistant directors (along with fiscal affairs) felt that these decisions should reflect the revenue-generating capacities of a proposal — if a project fit the institution's general strategy and could "make money" either in the short or the medium term, then it should be considered favorably. This viewpoint is not surprising, of course, given that the basic job of these assistant directors was to formulate requests from chiefs and department heads for new programs, personnel, and equipment into formal proposals that were financially justified and justifiable to fiscal affairs and the hospital's chief operating officer (COO). However, as one assistant director pointed out, financial benefit to the hospital did not in itself tip the scales: "The hospital wouldn't approve everything I asked for that makes money, because they're risk averse."

The hospital's chief executive officer (CEO), on the other hand, had to consider Oak Memorial's strategic position in relation both to other hospitals affiliated with the same medical school and to other large urban institutions in the city. Consequently, from this perspective, the issue for Oak Memorial was primarily one of its image as a vibrant institution with respected programs and physicians.

The danger in pursuing an exclusively prestige-oriented strategy, in the eyes of the lower-echelon administrators, was that financial considerations received too little attention. There was a tendency, as one of them put it, "to give away the ship without consulting the troops." The divergence in emphasis led in particular to tension within the administration over the issue of "dowries" for incoming chiefs of service.[2]

The different permutations involved in the complex set of intraadministration interests were best capsulized in the following comments by an assistant director:

> The dental unit here won't ever grow too large because it doesn't have teaching and research, but it will survive because it makes money. To survive, a program has to contribute one of the three: teaching, research, or money. Things were somewhat looser in the past, but the financial situation is so difficult that a new program must also break even on a full-cost basis before it could be started up now. Except if the chief of medicine or surgery wanted something badly, then he could have it on a direct-cost, break-even basis. I can think of one example of a program that is hard to manage because of conflict in the power structure, yet it got off the ground because it filled a competitive need and the push was from the CEO and the COO.

This is not to argue that either party to this differing perception of priorities was against continued institutional growth per se. Indeed, Oak Memorial had grown rapidly in the past ten years, and most members of the administration — like the chiefs of service — hoped to continue as rapid a pace of development as possible.

Interactions within the Medical Staff

The medical staff at Oak Memorial appeared to be a fairly cohesive unit when observed by those outside. There was a tendency among the hospital's administrators, as described above, to view the service chiefs as proxies for the medical staff and, in turn, to respond to them as a unified group. This impression of a unified stance led by a well-integrated set of leaders, while accurate in the formal sense, belied another set of interactions within the medical staff. These interactions, which were themselves related to issues of relative power and resource control, were subdivided into four categories: interactions among service chiefs, interactions within a service between its chief and his subchiefs, interactions between full-time salaried and part-time physicians, and interactions between attending physicians and the house staff (residents and interns).

INTERACTIONS AMONG SERVICE CHIEFS

Interactions among service chiefs were highly supportive on some occasions and highly competitive on others. One chief, for example, noted that he would seek support from his colleagues before "taking on" the CEO. Several second-echelon administrators confirmed that tendency, noting that sometimes two or more chiefs might explicitly decide to pursue a particular change of interest to them both. In such a situation, in the words of one administrator, "Prima facia it seems that something has been worked out. For example, the chief of radiology and the chief of orthopedic surgery seem to have made an arrangement to obtain a portable fluoroscopic device in the operating room for the chief of radiology. The chief of radiology, in turn, supported the chief of orthopedic surgery for renovations, which was of course part of the chief of orthopedics' dowry." This administrator noted that, similarly, a chief will often solicit support from his colleagues for a particular project: "The great tactic is to have colleagues say that you need a certain machine. You get a copy of the letter with a capital budget request."

The more competitive interactions among service chiefs at Oak Memorial appeared to involve direct resource allocation. As described by the chief of orthopedic surgery, the chief of medicine, the chief of surgery, and the chief of neurology, among others, these clashes tended primarily to be over dollar support and research space. Moreover, the relative ability of a chief to obtain his perceived needs reflected a complex mixture of prestige, size, and revenue, with resources flowing most readily to services that ranked high on all three criteria.

One technique Oak Memorial's senior administrators often used to mitigate these difficulties was to promise one of the competing chiefs he would receive his funds or space in a following year. This in effect created additional multiyear budgetary commitments so as to relieve resource pressures in the current year. The technique had been particularly effective in getting chiefs to surrender some of their present space for an incoming chief's dowry, often in return for the promise of replacement space upon completion of an anticipated new building. Oak Memorial's chief of surgery, for instance, noted two instances in which surgery had relinquished space under such conditions. In the first, he said, "We gave up some research space to pathology, in return for space in the new research building." Although this was to be a temporary situation, the chief commented that this was so only "if you call three years temporary." Surgery, among several other services, also gave up space to the new chief of medicine, though here the motives were a bit more complicated: "We gave up some space to medicine to recruit new subchiefs, but sometimes your department gains something here. The inability of medicine to recruit new subchiefs of cardiology and gastroenterology had hurt our department. The program we attracted was so good that we were willing to give up the space."

Oak Memorial's continued growth over the past ten years had clearly softened certain potential conflicts between service chiefs over available resources. Not only had there been a regularly increasing amount of space to allocate, but also there were often substantial new capital equipment budgets associated with these new facilities. The advantage of this growth to the anesthesiology service, for instance, was apparent. In the words of its chief, "I was told I would do okay for seven years—that is the life expectancy of the biomedical equipment. However, because we built a new building (some six years after I arrived), with eleven new operating rooms, we got entirely new equipment. Thus the new building made it administratively easier to get the department reequipped. Now too [some seven years later] we're having a new building."

In sum, conflict between chiefs over resources at Oak Memorial was often muted if not eliminated both by the ability of the hospital's senior administrators to use multiyear budgeting and by the continued growth in the hospital's facilities. Both mechanisms effectively enabled senior administrators to enlarge the available resource pie and thus to deflate what might otherwise have been considerably more intense competition among the service chiefs.

INTERACTIONS WITHIN SERVICES

The second area of intramedical relationships, within a service between its chief and his subchiefs, was much more hierarchical. Not only did the service chief hire the subchiefs, he retained almost total control over their ability to make administrative decisions. As the new chief of medicine obliquely phrased it, "With anyone I try to hire, as a chief, I try to keep as much flexibility as possible." In practical terms, this hierarchical chief/subchief relationship required subchiefs to obtain the permission of their service chief before they could seek programs, funds, faculty, or space from the administration. As one chief noted of a particular new program, "The individual who was particularly interested in this project worked with the department's administrative assistant [to write up a proposal], and I approved it."

This requirement to obtain prior approval was frustrating at times, particularly for growth-oriented subchiefs. One subchief, for instance, spoke bluntly about the problems it generated for him: "This leads to the big frustration for me: I don't know what's going on in this hospital except through my chief; if he says 'you can't have it,' there's no recourse."

Elaborating upon these difficulties, this same subchief explained the practical effects of this decision-making structure: "If I need space, I can't have it without my chief's permission. Space is a huge problem. I can't verify it without going to my chief; I have to make the assumption that he is being honest with me when he tells me what the status of things is in the hospital, and I do make that assumption." As this subchief summarized his perception of his situation, "My chief can do whatever he wants with space. In my professional life, he's the most powerful person."

Oak Memorial's neurosurgical subchief devised a somewhat unusual strategy to deal with his lowered status in the resource-commanding pecking order. Faced with what he perceived to be the absence of necessary clinical programs as well as adequate beds and equipment to pursue either patient care or teaching, he opted not to fight to obtain new resources but to concentrate nearly exclusively on research. In part his decision was made easier by his belief that there was an oversupply of surgeons in his specialty, but the logic of his solution remained one of professional realignment. As he described his approach, "The wise fox has several holes. You can use bottlenecks to do other things. My initial strategy was to control clinical activities by accepting the bottleneck of resources. I learned this by watching the ploys of several deans. More important, I have converted the problems of inadequate resources and an oversupply of neurosurgeons into an opportunity to do fundamental laboratory research."

The more standard response to the perceived subordinate role of a subchief was to seek a strategy which would increase his[3] power vis-à-vis his chief and the hospital administrators. One subchief with considerable clinical responsibility settled upon seeking control of the budget for his area. As he phrased his approach, "I'm not asking for divisional or department status, although this may develop, but I'm trying to establish my need to have control over the budget. I want the whole deal presented to me; how does the whole thing work, the nature of the beast. I want to be involved in the [capital and operating budgets] from the beginning."

Perhaps the most instructive demonstration of the nature of chief/subchief interactions at Oak Memorial, as well as about the entire process by which its chiefs and senior administrators develop new programs, was the experience of its kidney transplant subchief. As he described his experience: "The chief of surgery had brought me here because he wanted to start transplants here, but I had to go after my own grants to set the program up after I got here. . . . There was no way I could have gotten a freestanding unit here — they didn't have the beds or the space. Plus the administration was supportive because it didn't require a big program."

There was a four-year lag, however, before the first transplant operation was performed, until the hospital's dialysis facilities could be expanded: "The reason it took so long was that dialysis was weak here — we had only one machine. We needed a standard dialysis program; that's a much bigger commitment that had to be worked out because it requires space for machines and beds." Dialysis, though, was the responsibility of the department of medicine, and thus this subchief found himself forced to push his own chief to motivate the chief of medicine so that such a unit could be established: "I did this mainly by complaining that things were going slowly; I complained to my chief and he kept saying to me, 'don't worry, they'll do it.'" In the view of this subchief, Oak Memorial's administration had a primarily prestige-related reason to have him available, ready to do transplants, once the new dialysis program was in place: "The hospital wanted me aboard, to keep me busy, doing research, waiting for the time when a transplant program could start up. They wanted me here if they wanted to get their image up since they needed transplants." Ultimately, the new dialysis unit was established after a wealthy benefactor was found to underwrite the unit's capital costs, and the hospital's transplant service began shortly thereafter.

One related issue about which this subchief was uncertain was the effect of the then-impending decision of the federal Medicare program to pay for the costs of renal dialysis. Although he described the dialysis unit as "a big money maker; it makes scads of money," he commented that he did not know "whether that affected the hospital's decision to go into dialysis." In this regard, however, the CEO disagreed, saying, "his vision is grossly untrue. It never was nor is 'a big money maker.'"

Nevertheless, in the instance of this surgical subchief, there was the need to move not simply one but two service chiefs in order to obtain the desired program, yet the subchief's primary leverage was only that of complaint to his own chief. In this respect the hierarchical character of chief/subchief interactions was clearly illuminated.

The chief executive officer, however, sought to put the issue of chief/subchief relationships into its broader organizational perspective: "Since the chief of service is accountable for the entire service, it follows that he must have control over the allocation of resources to all subchiefs.

Many physicians cannot appreciate the distinction between professional autonomy and administrative autonomy."

INTERACTIONS BETWEEN FULL-SALARIED AND PART-TIME PHYSICIANS

The root cause of the tension between full-salaried and part-time physicians at Oak Memorial was the different emphasis on each group's activities. Salaried physicians tended to concentrate primarily on the more prestige-related activities, particularly research and publication, while part-timers placed most of their efforts on patient care. As one part-time physician bluntly presented his side of the issue, "When I went to medical school, the object was to take care of patients, not to do research. . . . In terms of patient care, these full-time people here see one or two or three patients, and they don't come in for emergencies." This part-time physician felt that the structure of power at Oak Memorial was based only on forms of prestige based on research and teaching and that patient-related forms of prestige were not highly valued. He phrased his view as follows: "Even though part-timers fill beds, they have little power in a teaching hospital. In community hospitals, physicians who fill beds have tremendous prestige, because they do fill beds. Part-timers are the people we honor at medical school, but they have no power in the teaching hospital. They're like a great slave, honored but subservient." This physician summarized this full-time/part-time tension with the contention that "essentially, the full-time heads of departments speak to themselves, and the question becomes, How will the generals plan for the privates?"

From the perspective of the service chiefs, part-timers were a two-sided issue. On the one hand, they brought patients, revenue, and often teaching capabilities to Oak Memorial. On the other hand, however, the chiefs tended to perceive part-timers as a vestigial remnant of a passing era. This ambivalence is perhaps best conveyed by the fact that, in the recent past, the chiefs of both surgery and medicine at Oak Memorial had sought to place all their hospital-based physicians in a full-time salaried relationship, but in both instances the resistance had been too strong for them to succeed. The position of the service chiefs concerning the role of private physicians can perhaps be summarized by the comments of Oak Memorial's new chief of medicine, first about his preceding appointment and then about Oak Memorial: "As against Oak Memorial, fewer than 2 percent of the beds at [his prior institution] were filled by privates. That was always a full-time hospital basically. And I didn't touch the role of the privates when I went there. There are no more than there were; however, they haven't been fired either. I was basically letting them retire with dignity and grace. With regard to the role of privates at Oak Memorial, I want to be sure that their quality is high, since they fill 55 percent of the hospital's beds. Moreover, I think they bring something special to the hospital besides patients."

INTERACTIONS BETWEEN ATTENDING PHYSICIANS AND HOUSE OFFICERS

The relationship between attending physicians and house officers is the last form of intramedical staff interactions at Oak Memorial. Here the nature of the relationship is rigidly hierarchical, indeed for a teaching institution classically so. Moreover, the division of clinical responsibilities among attending physicians, residents, and interns had direct cost containment implications for the hospital as a whole.

The driving characteristic of this particular subset of physician relationships at Oak Memorial was a concern with professional reputation and peer respect. One second-echelon administrator provided a lucid overview of the resource allocation implications for the hospital of the rather intricate set of teaching-hospital protocols:

> The house staff doesn't think about costs; they are worried about their performance as evaluated by their attending. No matter how fancy or costly the procedure, it's just a piece of clinical data for the resident. Attendings don't, I think, actually function as the primary caregiver—they are teachers. Essentially the intern does the scutwork, and on occasion orders procedures, but not much of the decision making. The resident does the conceptual work as to how the case will be managed. Each attending has his own regimen as to how much he'll let the resident do. With regard to rounds, the intern may present the case, but just the facts, not a decision tree. The resident comments on the case and suggests the course of action. The resident has to be sure that he doesn't look bad in front of his team, when the attending criticizes him and says, "Why didn't you do such-and-such a test? How can you make this decision without it?"

This perception of the intricate connection between clinical work, teaching, professional approval, and resource allocation was confirmed by Oak Memorial's chief of pathology. Commenting on the key role of the house staff in ordering laboratory tests, he noted, "This type of use is basically resident controlled, although attending physicians will make major decisions. Moreover, on many but not all services, clinic or nonprivate patients will have even major decisions made by the chief resident." Given the clear influence of attending physicians over house officers' future careers, there was a very strong tendency for residents and interns to utilize their ordering capacity to impress their supervisors. Moreover, house officers also recognized the importance of suppressing whatever tensions might emerge in their relationships with senior physicians. As one part-time physician noted, "Residents know if they fly off the handle at the chief of medicine it's suicide, but if you do it against a part-timer, it's not so serious."

In sum, then, despite the clearly dominant role of the service chiefs within the medical staff at Oak Memorial, there remained a series of internal interactions among physicians that could affect both the position of the medical staff as a whole and also the level of quality and resource efficiency found in the hospital's capital and operating activities. Although the external facade was smooth, beneath it lay considerable ferment.

Interactions between Medical Staff and Support Staff

At Oak Memorial, as in any hospital, the predominant focus of physician interaction with the support staff was the nursing service. And again, as in most other hospitals, physician/nurse interactions exhibited various tensions.

Precisely because nursing was a strong service at Oak Memorial, well respected both within and outside the hospital, the conflict was both greater and more openly acknowledged than might be the case elsewhere. One second-echelon nursing administrator analyzed the situation as follows: "There are two basic issues with nursing. The first is the need to develop relations with the physicians; they're not the enemy. The second is that nursing must be in an assertive position; the physician is new to collaboration, and the nurse must show the physician how to make that work. I hold the expectation that physicians are colleagues, not enemies." This nursing administrator explained that what was required was not particularly complicated: "It's not a sophisticated process; it just means that a physician can't blow up and scream, and that if a physician exhibits unacceptable behavior then you as a nurse have to confront. The key issue is in nurses confronting physicians directly."

Two recent examples were offered to illustrate the issues involved in physician/nurse tensions. Both, it should be noted, concerned patient-care decisions that physicians traditionally had considered inviolably theirs. The first, as described by another nursing director at Oak Memorial, addressed questions of physicians' orders: "The nurse is responsible to the patient and to the family. Nowhere do we say that the nurse is responsible to the physician. Physicians write orders, but if we don't agree with them we don't carry them out. Nurses on the open heart unit, for example, know what orders for medication should be, and they will call and ask a physician if they don't think a particular order is correct. There are a lot of interns and residents here who are new and who are grateful to have a nurse who can prevent them from making mistakes."

The second focused on nursing's perception of a conflict between physicians' orders and the nurse's function of patient education: "If a patient has a temperature after surgery and if the patient asks what the temperature reads, the nurse can tell the patient. The chief of surgery has written orders saying that the nurse should not tell the patient, and we ignore them. This is an example of one of the biggest issues between nurses and physicians. Nurses maintain that a patient has a right to know, and the physician maintains that physicians have the right to decide what the patient is told. This is really a question of a nurse's right to educate, and of the patient's right to learn about central issues from the nurses." This nursing administrator noted that the second conflict was one that was unlikely ever to be resolved at Oak Memorial: "This temperature thing will never come to a head. Here the administrator doesn't generally side with the physicians, as it traditionally has been done elsewhere, so the outcome is not a foregone conclusion." Summarizing the effect of these and other physician/nurse issues for the hospital overall, this nursing administrator suggested that there was an inherent structural difficulty owing to the nature of patient care: "Hospitals are never black and white; there's a huge gray area, and the nurses and physicians are caught in that. The more patient education nurses do, the bigger the gray area gets."

From the physicians' perspective, many of the tensions between the medical staff and nursing arose from nursing's desire to extend its zone of authority. This perception suffused the comments of a number of physicians, despite their professed respect for the quality and capabilities of the nursing service at Oak Memorial. One junior physician best capsulized this attitude when he contended that "Nurses want the independent decision-making power. You can call it 'this is wanting to be physicians,' whatever. It's basically a rebound phenomenon — nurses have been historically downtrodden, so now they're not going to let any doctor tell them what to do." This physician suggested that the structure of this conflict did not portent well for the future: "I think that all this will get worse rather than better. Looking at the nursing shortage, they're dissatisfied with bedside nursing. They want to become educators or they want to work in the ICU, because they don't have any power at the bedside. But I see a lack in bedside nurses because they want more power, rather than just doing the job that needs to be done at the bedside."

Again, the chief executive officer viewed the nursing issue in a somewhat broader perspective: "Clearly, the physician quoted had little concept of primary nursing as it is practiced at Oak Memorial. Nurses are *accountable* to the chief of nursing and not to physicians, but their accountability includes following the doctor's orders, within the limits of accountability dictated by their professional judgment."

In sum, then, there was a broad recognition among both medical and nursing staffs at Oak Memorial that fundamental decision-making issues were in dispute between them. While there was a general sense that there were more cooperative efforts to resolve these conflicts now than there had been in the past, in the final analysis there was a strong belief that resolution of the fundamental basis of this dispute was not likely in the near future. Yet, in the words of the chief executive officer, "from the patient's viewpoint, nursing at Oak Memorial was usually perceived as several cuts above nursing that the patient had received elsewhere."

Conclusions

The character of the chiefs of service's interactions along each of the three dimensions — with administrators, with other chiefs and physicians, and with the hospital's support staff — can be summarized in terms of three key aspects of Oak Memorial's present situation. First, the fundamental axis of decision-making authority within the institution lay in the relation between the service chiefs and the hospital's senior administrators. Second, the central decision-related incentive was a predominant concern, on the part of both chiefs and senior administrators, with institutional prestige, followed by a secondary concern at all levels (though most strongly expressed by second-level administrators) with financial issues. Third, second-echelon or assistant administrators played a vital role in expediting or delaying resource allocation.

CHAPTER 6
Programmatic Decision Making at Peninsula Community Hospital

The rather complex programmatic decision-making process that existed at Peninsula Community Hospital can be viewed first in light of some general decision-making criteria and then in terms of several program initiatives. As will be seen, a central issue is the "fit" between clinical and financial concerns.

Decision-Making Criteria

Programmatic decision making at Peninsula Community Hospital reflected the fact that the hospital's programs were in constant flux. At any given time, a wide variety of delivery options were competing for financial resources. By evaluating those recent options that were implemented easily and those that were not, as well as the way options were considered, one can obtain a deeper understanding of the underlying incentives that explain the actual resource-allocation process. More particularly, a careful comparison of proposals that were implemented easily with those that were not suggests that two fundamental forces drove decision making at Peninsula. As might be anticipated, one was the hospital administration's major concerns; the other was the central concerns of the medical staff.

ADMINISTRATIVE CONCERNS

The dominant concern for the hospital's chief administrator was the financial survival of the hospital itself. Faced with an increasingly difficult financial climate both in terms of tighter regulation and reimbursement limits and in terms of heightened competition for patients, in evaluating program proposals the chief administrator looked closely at their ability to generate new revenue for the hospital. All requests for new services or for improvement to existing services, capital or noncapital in orientation, were evaluated primarily in terms of their effect on the hospital's bottom line.

The first tenet of the hospital's "survival strategy" — as one senior administrator described it — was to restructure the organization into two sister corporations: one for activities subject by statute to regulatory and reimbursement review, the other meant to pursue spinoffs of the hospital's traditional activities. A for-profit operation was being set in motion during the study period but had not yet begun to generate any substantial revenue for the hospital. As conceived, this for-profit endeavor was to engage initially in such medically related but off-budget endeavors as an occupational health program aimed at nearby industry and the construction and management of a new medical arts building on the building grounds. It was not intended, at that time, to enter into any activities completely unrelated to the hospital's primary (i.e., medical) mission.

The second, complementary tenet of the strategy was to improve the revenue flow from in-hospital medical activities. The strategic means to this increased revenue flow can be divided into three elements: the addition of selected new services and programs within the hospital; the recruitment of additional physicians for selected services; and the reorganization of several existing arrangements with salaried physicians into volume-sensitive group practices.

From the administration's perspective, physicians' practice concerns were viewed as not particularly helpful in the pursuit of the hospital's revenue objectives. Indeed, administrators tended to have a rather split view of Peninsula's medical staff. On the one hand, some tended to see physicians as little aware of the financial implications their pet projects had for the hospital. As one administrator phrased it, "physicians think the amount of money available is infinite." Yet on the other hand, the administrators recognized that they held a "high mortality job" and that one common way to lose it was to lose the confidence of the medical staff. Consequently, they felt it essential to devise an overall institutional strategy that could successfully restrain the physicians' desire for expansion unrelated to the hospital's short-term survival yet that would not alienate the medical staff. The administrators felt further constrained by the rotation of the chiefs of service, which meant that, as one put it, "there's no institutional memory" in the clinical departments, and discussions about a particular project often had to begin anew upon the election of a new chief.

PHYSICIANS' CONCERNS

In contrast to the administrators, the primary concern of Peninsula's attending physicians was not for the hospital's revenues, but for their own individual or group medical practices. Indeed, since the pathologists, radiologists, and anesthesiologists described themselves as fully dependent for the success of their careers upon the approval of the clinical staff, one can conclude that the fundamental motivation of all physicians at Peninsula was, first, the protection, and second, the further development and expansion of their own medical practices.

This central concern of physicians for the health of their practices expressed itself, as one would expect, in myriad forms. Indeed, this force was so dominant that it infused almost every resource decision that Peninsula's attending physicians made. These physician-determined decisions extended across a broad spectrum of the hospital's activities, from patient satisfaction (e.g., whether ordering a telemetry monitoring unit might impress a patient's family), to concern that intervention by social services in a case of child abuse might harm the physician's relationship with the family, to more major issues about the need to restructure physicians' responsibility in the emergency room. From a more programmatic perspective, the issues ranged from adding a body scanner to the clinicians' diagnostic armamentarium to developing an entirely new clinical program (sports medicine). Whether negatively expressed (as fear of inroads into their present practices) or positively expressed (as decisions on a particular practice-building program or program change) it is fair to say that concern for their practices dominated most physicians' decision-making behavior at Peninsula.

It is important to stress that this concern for protecting and developing their practices was not solely financial. To be sure, personal income did figure in these practice-related decisions; however, the issue often involved long-run rather than short-run considerations. More important, financial motives in any form were clearly only one of several major incentives that generated this practice orientation. For example, a key element for both attending and hospital-based physicians was the respect of their professional peers. A number of physicians spoke of the importance of being accepted by their medical colleagues, not solely for patient referrals but also in terms of professional self-respect. Moreover, even highly patient-related issues, like the size of one's practice and the extent of one's referral network, were important for the peer recognition and professional prestige they conferred. Indeed, in a number of instances a clinician's decision on a major practice-related matter appeared to be determined as much by concern for professional stature as by either short- or long-term revenue.

From the physicians' perspective, the administration at Peninsula appeared not to understand the fundamental requirements for high-quality care. As one internist put it, "Basically, the administration is supposed to be just supplying the necessary equipment and personnel to support state of the art medicine." Consequently, many physicians expressed considerable frustration with the administration's revenue priorities. The same clinician continued, "Anything that is done takes years and years . . . they have to be sure they're going to make money." A number of physicians also expressed intense concern at what they felt was a tendency to sit on problems and requests rather than resolving them. One surgeon summarized this perception with the statement that the administration's style was "to recognize the problem, to bring in outside help, to discuss it at all levels, and then let the problem dissipate — not solve it, let it dissipate." Or as one of the hospital-based physicians put it, a bit more cynically, "this may be a pretty standard technique, letting things drag; I get the feeling they do it as a regular technique here."

Finally, most physicians felt strongly that the continued turnover of chief administrators proved their contention that it was the medical staff, not the administration, that had the hospital's best interests at heart. Peninsula had had three chief administrators in the past five years, and some of the more long-standing clinicians said there had been seven over the past twenty years. As a result, physicians saw the chief administrator as someone who appears, makes some rapid changes, and then leaves the hospital — and their practices — with the consequences. A number of physicians mentioned that the lack of a stable administration made it difficult to negotiate a proposed project to completion, since it was continually necessary to begin again with a new chief administrator.

Program Initiatives

For ease of discussion, these program initiatives can be divided into four categories: new services, reorganization of existing services, capital equipment, and renovations. Despite the differing levels of reimbursement, revenue, and practice-related implications of these four groups, the key factors that drive Peninsula's decision-making process were both apparent in and common to them all.

NEW SERVICES

Of the eleven proposed new programs or services identified at Peninsula Community Hospital, six were particularly illustrative of the constellation of forces and incentives that affected whether a proposed service would be implemented. These six were (in no particular order) an outpatient psychiatry clinic, an inpatient dialysis service, a sports medicine program, a telemetry unit, an endoscopy service, and a midwife program.

Outpatient Psychiatry Clinic

The impetus to set up an outpatient mental health clinic initially came from the chief of psychiatry, but the suggestion was rapidly supported by the hospital's chief administrator. At the time, the psychiatry chief had a number of new program proposals, all of which would expand available services or increase overall patient volume. The outpatient clinic was, as he put it, "on my shopping list; however, I didn't expect to get it for five years because the private practice physicians are leery of clinics."[1] Faced with something of a revolt over this issue, the chief sought to convince the private physicians that they would gain referrals from the new clinic rather than losing existing patients to psychologists and social workers on the clinic's staff. To further ensure their acquiescence, the chief brought the private clinicians into the clinic itself, allowing each to contribute one-half day per week, for which they were not paid but did receive referrals.

Moreover, the clinic was structured to provide short-term treatment exclusively, and those clinic patients who were covered by private insurance were informed on their first visit that they could elect to be evaluated by a private psychiatrist. These privately insured patients were told that this alternative course could be advantageous should the patient require additional therapy later, since private practitioners usually would remain associated with the hospital for the remainder of their professional careers. These caveats and constraints were sufficient to win the clinic's acceptance by the private psychiatrists.

The chief administrator at Peninsula also favored a rapid start-up for the outpatient mental health clinic. The hospital's for-profit sister corporation was initiating its new occupational health program, and that program required just such a clinic setting for employees who might seek counseling or short-term therapy. Moreover, the absence of any major capital outlay, the operating structure of the clinic, and the occupational health program's insurance coverage ensured that the clinic would be financially successful.

Thus, in large part as the result of this confluence of motivations among the chief of psychiatry, the private psychiatrists, and the chief administrator, an outpatient mental health clinic was soon opened on the hospital grounds, staffed by four new hospital-salaried full-time workers.

Inpatient Dialysis Service

The impetus for an inpatient dialysis unit came from a relatively young general surgeon on the medical staff at Peninsula. He explained the need for such a unit in terms of his own practice: "There are a certain number of people in a large surgical practice who go into renal shock and renal failure. I'm trained to take care of sick people, and I need this unit to take care of them, to support these patients. . . . It meant that they could stay here, and they could be treated by their own physician."

This surgeon's efforts to get inpatient dialysis began with an invitation to a nephrologist from one of the nearby teaching hospitals to join the medical staff. The nephrologist subsequently obtained a donated dialysis machine and wrote up the necessary justification to obtain administrative approval for both space and staffing. At the time of the study, although the dialysis unit was strictly for acute inpatient care, it had generated enough patients both to be financially viable and to require additional dialysis nurses.[2]

In this instance the confluence of incentives among this particular surgeon, the nephrologist, and the hospital administration produced a fairly rapid installation and had the potential to generate the expansion of an inpatient dialysis program at the hospital.

Sports Medicine

The third new program proposal at Peninsula was sports medicine. The primary moving force behind this service addition was the chief of orthopedic surgery, who felt that such a service was necessary to ensure that athletic injuries at the elementary- and secondary-school levels received the same treatment as those at the college level.

This chief set out to design a program that would avoid the errors made by sports medicine programs in other hospitals. To do so, he used personal funds to visit a number of existing programs, touring their facilities and interviewing the staff. During this same period he met with Peninsula's chief administrator regularly to ensure that the program would be properly designed for reimbursement purposes. One of the major advantages of the proposal, in this physician's eyes, was that it could be implemented almost entirely with equipment the hospital already owned. The total new capital investment for the program, he calculated, would be only eighteen thousand dollars. When the proposal was sufficiently developed, he presented it to his department, giving them a host of specifics such as the fees to be charged and the controls that would be placed on such abuses as unnecessary surgery. When he finally presented the proposal to the board of trustees for approval, he could give them every essential detail. As he put it, "I went to the board with a complete package deal."

Peninsula's chief administrator was extremely pleased with this sports medicine proposal in every respect. Not only could it be implemented with minimal initial outlay, but it was a reimbursable service that did not require a certificate of need.[3] Furthermore, as the administrator enthusiastically noted, "it's a great marketing tool."

In this third instance, then, there was again a confluence of practice, revenue, and practical logistic interests between the chief of orthopedic surgery and the chief administrator that led to the proposed program's rapid adoption.

Telemetry Unit

The fourth program proposal at Peninsula had a somewhat more difficult history. In the three preceding examples, the "fit" between the practice concerns on the initiating physician and the revenue concerns of the administrators had ensured rapid agreement and implementation. The telemetry unit, however, involved a constellation of incentives that were rather less clearly in concert, and consequently the approval and implementation process was substantially more extended.

A telemetry unit might best be described as a coronary care unit (CCU) stepdown. Through a system of mobile transmitters, it enables a physician to monitor a patient's vital signs electronically without placing that patient in the highly intensive — and very expensive — CCU. Thus a telemetry unit provides a post-CCU way station before the patient is moved onto a regular floor, freeing up a CCU bed for a more acutely ill patient. It also functions as an alternative placement for those patients who were, as Peninsula's chief of medicine put it, "not 100 percent CCU patients."

At the time of the study, the telemetry unit had been under consideration for some four years. One of the unit's strongest proponents, a senior physician in the department of medicine, had arranged for one of his patients to donate the funds necessary to purchase the monitoring equipment, but it had remained in storage. Indeed, before the unit could finally go into operation, that equipment had to be sent back to the manufacturers to be retested. On several occasions plans were set in motion to begin the necessary renovations on the designated medical/surgical floor, but each time the process failed to come to fruition.

This lack of resolution was particularly evident in contrast to what had been a very rapid change in the same floor's designation just before the initial telemetry request. At that time, most of the beds were designated for a low-intensity progressive care unit, providing the minimal supervision required for patients waiting to be discharged. The pressure from attending physicians to fill these beds with medical/surgical patients became so intense, however, particularly during the winter when the hospital tended to be full, that within a rather short time the progressive care unit was disbanded and the floor given over for general medical/surgical admissions.

The subsequent effort to transform some of these new medical/surgical beds into a telemetry unit, however, though approved by the administration, dragged on for a period some physicians found interminable. Moreover, no one seemed to know the reason for the delay — the chief of medicine, for example, said, "I can't say the administration was delaying, but the unit was delayed for some reason." There was the additional complication that the hospital had three new chief administrators during this four-year period.

The advantages of establishing a telemetry unit, as noted above, were somewhat less uniform for all parties than those in the previous three examples. The medical staff believed a telemetry unit would enable them to monitor more patients electronically. Indeed, the incentive to order such monitoring was strong enough that the chief of medicine felt he had to institute fairly strict rules on the new unit's use: "I know from experience in the medical department that everyone wants a monitor. Some physicians generally abuse the system, and I felt they would abuse this system unless there were some kind of rules. Why do they abuse? It could be for income purposes; every human being is looking for income, especially when you're young and starting out a practice. It's very difficult to determine."

Despite this combination of quality-of-care and practice-building incentives, however, the pressure from most attending physicians to open a telemetry unit was not intense. Indeed, some physicians noted that the push to have a telemetry unit largely reflected the desires of only "some" of those in the medical department. One likely reason for this lower priority, of course, was that those beds designated for this new unit were already available for medical/surgical admissions, and thus the disadvantage of opening the new unit was that it would decrease medical/surgical bed capacity with a service that could be provided elsewhere (in the CCU).

Establishing a telemetry unit was not of immediate importance to Peninsula's administration either. As the chief of medicine noted, "this isn't a high earner." Moreover, despite the carrot of donated equipment, the hospital would have had to bear substantial renovation costs as well as the cost of training nurses to run the monitors. Last, for a hospital that already had a CCU, there was little additional patient flow or marketing value to be gained from a telemetry unit. Indeed, according to the chief administrator, "There were several barriers to rapid implementation of the telemetry unit: first, the equipment on hand had to be evaluated and upgraded; second, a new director of engineering had to be hired [and was]; and third, a complicated antenna system had to be installed throughout the hospital."

In sum, then, although there was a substantial practice incentive on the part of attending physicians and considerable pressure from several of them, the effect of administrative turnover coupled with logistic difficulties and low additional revenues to the hospital meant it took four years before the unit finally was in operation.

Endoscopy Suite

The next-to-last program proposal we will examine was an endoscopy room. This proposal had been under consideration for some years and had acquired a rather colorful history. When it was originally presented to the administrators, they questioned whether there was sufficient patient volume to justify a new facility. Despite their sense that their negative response had resolved the issue, the initiating surgeon nonetheless arranged for a former patient to donate funds to purchase equipment for the endoscopy room. These funds were channeled as a gift from a hospital-related charity group,[4] and the key physicians who wanted the new room believed that the administration had long since changed course and agreed to the new service. As the present chief of surgery explained the situation,

"The administration approved it, and it had to go to the finance committee of the board. This was done two years ago, or even three years ago." The chief administrator disagreed, stating emphatically, "Not so!"

There was palpable frustration among the physicians involved, however, because the service still was not in operation. The chief of surgery continued, "Although it's been promised for some time, we have never yet gotten the room. Originally we were told that one room had been set aside and that it was going to be made available; now we've been told that room will no longer be available and it will be somewhere else, but we don't know where."

When one looks at the differing incentives of the medical staff and the administration, it appears that in this case — as in that of the telemetry unit — there was a less than perfect "fit." The primary motivation of internists and surgeons who performed endoscopic procedures was, simply put, convenience. As the chief of surgery put it, "Why does a colonoscopist want a special room? Essentially and only because it's convenient for him, nothing else." The absence of an endoscopy suite required physicians to do these procedures in the operating room. This in turn meant, again in the words of the chief of surgery, "you need to schedule time in the OR, and as a result, since it's a minor operation, you get lousy times — late at night, early in the morning, etc." Additionally, because Peninsula's operating rooms were fully booked at that time, the availability of a specific endoscopy room would make it possible to perform more of these procedures.

The administration's motives regarding the endoscopy request remain a bit more obscure. In the eyes of several physicians, the only possible motive the administration could have was that it wanted to keep endoscopic procedures in the operating room because it generated higher reimbursement. As one surgeon summarized this view, "The hospital wants to keep the OR going for colonoscopies because it generates much greater revenue when they bill patients. The charges are in the hundreds for performing colonoscopy in the OR, whereas if you're just having a colonoscopy room, the charge is much less, under a hundred dollars in many hospitals."

Again, this assessment was at odds with that of the chief administrator, who responded, "This is absolutely not true! Space became the major problem because of the expansion of the emergency department. My belief is that the service can be built to answer a need." This administrative assessment was reinforced by suggestions from other senior administrators who felt that the service lacked sufficient patient volume to justify dedicated space, particularly since there was intense competition within the hospital for any available space.

Here, then, one can clearly conclude, much as in the case of the telemetry unit, that the physicians' practice incentives to have an endoscopy room were not sufficient to overcome the administration's hesitation to give this new service a high priority. In part the administration's hesitation appeared to be financially based.

Midwife Program

The last (and in some ways the most interesting) proposal for program change at Peninsula was to add midwifery to the obstetrical department's available services. Faced with a consistently low census in his department and the threat of closure by state regulatory agencies, the chief of obstetrics believed this new program would attract an additional segment of the population to the hospital's maternity service. As he described the proposal, "I'm thinking about bringing midwives here. There are two women who would like to use Peninsula, to bring their patients here. I know who they are; I provide backup service for them at this point now. I would like to set up a model program here, with birthing cottages, with these women running the program and with us in the department providing obstetrical backup."

The chief realized that this service addition would not be very popular with some obstetricians, however, since it was likely that they themselves would not gain additional patients through it. In fact, some obstetricians feared they might lose part of their existing practices: "There's resistance from some of the men on our present staff; they're afraid of losing patients."

The question of midwives, of course, raises the issue of competition from allied health professionals for obstetricians in much the same way that the introduction of psychologists in the outpatient mental health clinic raised the question for Peninsula's private psychiatrists. Although the proposed program's implementation might increase the maternity service's overall census, the lack of substantial support among some of the obstetrical staff suggested that the administration would face considerable resistance to this new program. Also, midwives at Peninsula, like most maternity services, were unlikely to generate any substantial revenue for the hospital.

As a result, although the hospital administration considered a midwife program a viable option and supported it, the interest level was not high for actually implementing the proposal. Moreover, there had been no significant pressure from the obstetrical department to counteract this apparent lack of interest.

REORGANIZATION OF EXISTING SERVICES

The types of incentives and motive forces that were dominant in the disposition of new program proposals also had a substantial influence on efforts to restructure existing services. In service reorganization, in fact, the competing concerns of the several occupational groups were more clearly delineated. Two prototypical examples of such reorganization encountered at Peninsula Community Hospital concerned the emergency room (ER) and the anesthesia department.

Emergency Room

There were several long-standing issues about physician staffing for the emergency room at Peninsula. These problems reflected the existing reimbursement arrangements for the ER, in which physicians' services were included as part of the hospital's Blue Cross reimbursement rather than being paid directly through Blue Shield.[5]

This Blue Cross reimbursement arrangement had a number of disadvantages in the eyes of both the hospital and the medical staff. First, the hospital had to pay ER physicians from its own Blue Cross payment. Second, this Blue Cross system required the physicians to negotiate a separate payment arrangement with the hospital. Worst of all, from the viewpoint of the medical staff, the existing system allowed the hospital the option—should it so decide—to hire separate full-time salaried physicians for the ER and also for its new industrial medicine program. There were thus not only financial issues but also critical practice considerations at stake here, since the number of salaried physicians could at some future time be expanded by the hospital to staff a full-time ambulatory clinic, which would of course directly compete for patients with the hospital's fee for service medical staff.

The resolution of this problem, developed by the same influential surgeon who had proposed the endoscopy suite, was to establish a separate, private corporation that would contract with the hospital for ER services. All members of the Peninsula medical staff who so desired could join the corporation and receive ownership shares. Furthermore, although physicians who were members of the private corporation would be allowed to provide off-hour or industrial medicine coverage, only members of the medical and surgical staff could admit patients.

This new arrangement appeared to be satisfactory to all parties. Peninsula's physicians provided coverage for the ER, which increased their own referrals, yet they did not fear losing patients who might visit the ER during off hours. Financially speaking, the physicians could now be paid through Blue Shield, which both increased their return and enabled the hospital to retain the entire Blue Cross payment. As the chief of surgery summarized the overall result of this new agreement, "this was potentially a revenue-producing area, which we have now managed to set up properly."

Although this instance was one of service reorganization rather than of a new program proposal, once again there was a clear confluence of medical staff and administration incentives that led in turn to an amicable and rapidly applied solution to the problem.

Anesthesia Department

The outcome of the second suggested service reorganization, concerning the hospital's contract with its anesthesiologists, was neither as clear-cut nor as rapid. The issue here was the terms of anesthesia's new group contract with the hospital. Under the existing arrangement, the anesthesiologists were salaried to the hospital; however, they now preferred to return to a fee for service structure (which had been the arrangement until some ten years before). Although anesthesia presented this change as an issue of practice independence, both the administration and other physicians perceived it as directly financial. As one surgeon summarized the common view, "Anesthesia now may want to go fee for service because they stand to make more money that way."

The administration supported the return to fee for service but saw the anesthesiologists as "resisting the effort." From the administration's perspective, however, the renegotiation of the anesthesia department's contract also raised the issue of off-hour staffing for the operating room — which anesthesia had resisted while on the salaried arrangement — and a related long-standing dispute between anesthesia and obstetrics over the absence of epidural anesthesia in the delivery room. Providing epidurals had become a rather contentious issue at the hospital. Despite the fact that the obstetrical service at Peninsula was clearly underutilized (indeed, there had been a recent regulatory effort to close the service down), anesthesia refused to provide what the chief of obstetrics described as "one of the most common and useful procedures." Moreover, as part of the same dispute, anesthesia has insisted upon "a protocol for their presence for delivery." In the words of the chief of obstetrics, "The issue for the anesthesiologists is basically time: they don't want to wait around. They've insisted, for example, that if they're involved in cesarean sections that they must be scheduled in advance like any other operation. Basically, most anesthesiologists don't like OB, because it's night service and you lose sleep." This problem between anesthesia and obstetrics had grown to the point where some members of the obstetrical department had threatened to move their practices if anesthesia did not become more responsive.

Finally, again tied to this issue of twenty-four-hour coverage, the administration felt that any new contract should contain a volume incentive to encourage full utilization of the hospital's operating rooms. The fundamental obstacle for the administration, however, was the hospital's reimbursement position. The same surgeon quoted above expressed the problem succinctly when he concluded that "the hospital may not want to give up the salary relationship because the hospital is making a lot of money by having the ability to keep the excess earnings."

At the time of the study, discussions over the anesthesia contract had been going on for more than a year, with no immediate resolution in sight. In this instance, consequently, quite unlike that of the emergency room reorganization, the various incentives of physicians and administrators were not at all in concert, and reaching agreement appeared difficult and time-consuming.

CAPITAL EQUIPMENT

The capital-intensive nature of inpatient care might lead one to expect a considerable number of proposals for capital-equipment acquisitions. Indeed, not only were there requests for specific pieces of equipment, but there were (as described above) various incidents in which donated capital equipment was used as leverage to obtain a new service. This section will concentrate on one highly indicative — and expensive — instance of capital-equipment acquisition, that of a body scanner.

The alignment of forces on the issue of the body scanner was a bit complicated owing to some competitive feelings over resources between the radiology and pathology departments. The initial request came from radiology, at the prodding of various members of the clinical staff. That the two like-sized hospitals on either side of Peninsula each had a body scanner in operation increased some internists' sense of urgency. By the period under study, the administration had agreed to purchase a body scanner and, in conjunction with two other hospitals, had filed a certificate of need application for a shared system.

The radiology department had attempted to design its initial proposal so that it would be financially attractive to the administration. In terms of operating budgets, radiology planned to train all its present technicians to run the new machine, so that there would be no additional personnel costs associated with its purchase. Radiology intended to arrange for outside investment capital to buy the body scanner for the group practice, which would in turn rent space for it from the hospital. This capital arrangement would also maximize the hospital's reimbursement return under then-existing regulations.

The administration had assented to radiology's proposal and had filed a certificate of need application for the machine. The status of this proposed capital addition at the time of the study was well summarized by the chief of radiology: "As far as the body scanner is concerned, that's purely a problem between the hospital and the state. As soon as we get a certificate of need, we will have it in."

The ease with which the administration and the proposing department agreed to acquire the body scanner belies a substantially less clear-cut situation in the eyes of both the administration and the medical staff. At least one member of the administration felt that the body scanner was not crucial to the hospital's competitive position because it already had the more vital head scanner. The administrator felt that the body scanner was being acquired only because of pressure from radiology. His interpretation, in turn, was supported not only by a second administrator, who perceived radiology as "the squeaky wheel," but also by several members of Peninsula's medical staff. In the words of the chief of medicine, "You really don't use the body scanner for emergencies, whereas for the head scan you need it for emergencies and it's hard to move patients. Thus the body scan is not such a big deal; it's not an emergency situation as with the head scan. We've lived without it for some time. If we had a body scan everyone would go first to that, and they wouldn't think of the easy, less expensive procedures, particularly if they were young and trained on the body scan."

Furthermore, there was direct pressure on the administration from another equally revenue-generating hospital-based department, pathology, to postpone any investment for the body scanner until funds had been committed to pathology's long-awaited space expansion. Pathology's project should be, in one pathologist's terms, "first on the runway." Another pathologist expressed his view of the problem as follows: "There has been some medical staff activity to get going on the body scanner; however, in a medical staff meeting we made it clear that we felt the pathology lab really had to have its space regardless whether the body scanner was or was not approved."

Thus, in this instance the pressures to acquire this piece of machinery were of varying intensity. Of the medical staff, radiology and some clinicians pushed very strongly for it, but other clinicians and the pathology department saw the body scanner as a mixed blessing. In turn, some members of the administration were also less than convinced of its necessity. Nonetheless, the administration had readily assented to the proposal and sought to fulfill it with dispatch, although to justify it they agreed to purchase the scanner in conjunction with two other hospitals in the area.

RENOVATIONS

The last of the four program categories under discussion is renovations to existing facilities. The proposed pathology department expansion has already been mentioned in connection with the body scanner and will not be pursued beyond noting that pathology had in fact been given the go-ahead by the administration and was awaiting approval of a certificate of need application. This section will examine another request, one that was not from a hospital-based department and was, indeed, quite the opposite in revenue-generating characteristics from requests by either radiology or pathology. This was a proposal from the department of obstetrics to renovate the hospital's labor rooms.

This proposed renovation was intended to complete the service's transformation to a modern family-centered program. It would entail some fifty thousand dollars for the purchase of birthing beds, more pleasant decor, and, most important, the remodeling of the existing large ward (divided only by curtains) into individual rooms.

Although construction was under way in early 1983, the decision to initiate it had taken what the chief of obstetrics considered an extended period. In reflecting on the process he commented, "I have a sense that the administration was putting pressure on us to bring up our census. I had a meeting with the administration about the construction project and then nothing happened for six months." Noting the obstetrical service's brush with closure a few years earlier, the chief concluded about the administration's attitude toward the renovation request: "I think they were waiting to see what was going to develop with the service — whether we were going to survive or not."

Summary

In general, the character of resource-related decision making at Peninsula Community Hospital can be summarized in four related points:

- The essential behavior incentives around which resource allocation turned were the administrators' concern with hospital revenue and need and the physicians' concern with their private practices.
- The fundamental decision-making axis ran between administrators and the medical staff.
- Other professional groups at the hospital, including the nursing staff and medical technicians, were not major actors in the hospital's decision making.
- The array of structural and functional decision-related levers strongly favored the medical staff; sooner or later, Peninsula's physicians usually got what they wanted.

CHAPTER 7
Programmatic Decision Making at Oak Memorial Medical Center

Oak Memorial Medical Center had a rather complex programmatic decision-making process, one that was seen quite differently by senior management, middle management, and service chiefs. In part, these differences reflected the three groups' relations with the hospital's department of fiscal affairs, and in part they were reflective of the hospital's overall power equilibrium.

Senior Management's Perspective

From the standpoint of Oak Memorial's senior administrators, the hospital's decision making took place within a highly effective administrative structure. After substantial effort, both middle- and lower-echelon administrators as well as chiefs of service were familiar with how the system was intended to function, and in the eyes of senior management everyone by and large adhered to the formal procedures.

Structurally speaking, the chiefs' primary point of access to the administration (at least in terms of requests for program changes or capital equipment) was through the assistant directors for their services. The role of an assistant director vis-à-vis a chief was as a facilitator and advocate — to develop a chief's request into a justifiable proposal. In the words of the chief operating officer (COO), the assistant directors "have a primary responsibility to facilitate and to support their chiefs. . . . We're not here to be the antagonists of the people who produce our products; we're here to make it easy for them to be effective and efficient." This perspective was in fact how the assistant directors themselves described their role within the hospital. As one put it, "I essentially work as an advocate and a resource for the chiefs."

Superimposed upon this formal layered administrative structure was a management philosophy of collegiality between the administrators and the chiefs. One central premise of this approach was a collaborative and consensus-oriented decision-making environment in which the chiefs shared, as the COO put it, the "team spirit." This entailed, primarily, a recognition by the administration that they ought not presume to treat the chiefs — or indeed any physician — as subordinates. The COO elaborated on this premise and its underlying philosophy as follows: "No boss/subordinate relationship exists between chiefs of service and administrators. We have to deal with each other on a collegial, negotiated basis. We try to foster a system of collegiality."

A second element of this collegial system, in the eyes of senior administrators, was that the chiefs could still come directly to the chief executive officer (CEO) with an issue. It is with respect to this element of the process in particular that the relationship of collegiality to the formal administrative structure becomes apparent: the CEO listens sympathetically but then suggests that the chiefs put their requests through the appropriate assistant directors. In the CEO's words, they "get the best of both worlds. They can get my ear, vent their spleen, but then we force them back into the administrative system."

Two additional aspects of this managerial approach deserve mention. The first revolves around the way senior management endeavors to openly discuss efforts by other institutions to recruit its chiefs. "We try to talk openly and candidly about offers we have had," according to the CEO. "To share this type of thing is symptomatic of the kind of collegial relationship we try to foster."

The second, more negatively construed aspect concerned the insistence of senior administrators that chiefs' threats of resignation would not deflect revenue-related determinations. In the words of the CEO, "On a day-to-day basis, there is no implied threat of 'if you don't do this, I'll leave.' One chief did it once, and I considered telling him 'I'll take you up on it.' It's not a unit of commerce around here. It's inappropriate."

The outcome of this administrative system, in the eyes of its primary designers and implementers, is an administrative decision-making process based largely on consensus. As the COO summarized what he considered to be the acid test of this management philosophy: "When we put the final budget out, I rarely hear cries of anguish from the trenches." The COO did suggest, however, that this consensus approach was predicated on the existence of sufficient funds for both operating and capital purposes. "Many administrators don't realize," he noted, "that to run an organization like this properly they are going to have to spend large sums of money." He also commented in this regard that "many institutions don't provide adequate funding for their capital-equipment budgets, and over time they are overwhelmed by obsolescence."

In the final analysis, however, Oak Memorial's senior management believed they had designed a fair and equitable administrative structure, one that met the chief's real needs while not becoming, in the words of one administrator, "a giveaway machine."

Middle Management's Perspective

There was some disagreement with this essentially positive assessment of how Oak Memorial's decision-making process worked. When one moved to the lower administrative echelons, the most common perception heard was, in fact, that the hospital administration placed few if any real constraints on the chiefs' demands. Indeed, lower-level administrators tended to agree strongly with the view of the chiefs themselves, which was that chiefs did in fact usually obtain whatever they set out to get.

From the perspective of the lower-echelon administrators, the central resource-allocation issue at Oak Memorial was not *whether* the chiefs of service had their demands met, but rather *how* and *when*. There was, first, the distinction between program and capital decisions that were generated "top down," in the form of critical "dowries" to incoming chiefs of service (of which more will be said shortly), and those generated "bottom up" by requests for changes from existing chiefs. These "bottom up" requests, in the words of one lower-echelon administrator, were classified into one of three categories: "far out or stupid ideas; good ideas that are legitimate and that we fund; good ideas we would like to do that we can't fund." In turn, this last, unfunded category "consists of two subcategories: programs that are not funded because they are too expensive, and programs that are approved but not funded *this year*." Summarizing the result of this allocation framework, the administrator concluded that decisions were ultimately based on a mixture of institutional strategy concerns and a strong need to keep the service chiefs satisfied: "Chiefs do get what they want, depending on the administration's view of how important it is. Importance is analyzed in terms of for institutional programs, for keeping a given chief happy, and for keeping a given chief on board."

This overarching role of the hospital's service chiefs in determining resource flow was apparent in numerous comments by lower-echelon administrators. Moreover, the second-echelon administrators' concerns extended beyond major resource questions to more mundane issues. In the rather revealing verbal shorthand of one, "The hospital has a rather laissez-faire attitude toward chiefs: senior administrators usually let the chiefs run their own show."

THE ISSUE OF DOWRIES

The attitude of Oak Memorial's senior administrators toward incoming chiefs' dowries was that they were a normal and necessary aspect of a teaching hospital. In the words of the COO, dowries were "required in order to successfully recruit in academic medicine." Indeed, the hospital's CEO argued that dowries made a direct, positive contribution to the hospital's growth and development: "Everyone recognizes that when you get a new generation that is looking to the future they'll come in with a lot of ideas. Thus it is inevitable that the vigor and growth and development of a service will take a quantum leap with a new chief. It wouldn't make sense not to provide a dowry for a new chief." Although the CEO did add the qualification that a dowry "has to follow program and it has to be realistic," his clear thrust was that the institution of the dowry had a beneficial effect on the hospital as a whole.

Quite unlike this perspective, the view of the lower-echelon administrators at Oak Memorial might best be described as apoplectic resignation — the apoplexy generated by the enormous drain on available resources created by such dowries. While the current concern revolved around commitments made to the new chief of medicine, several of these middle-rank administrators noted that in the past ten years Oak Memorial had given multimillion-dollar dowries to a number of new chiefs, including those of radiology and pathology, and sizable commitments had been made to other recently arrived chiefs. As one of the second-level administrators characterized the dowry system: "Each chief, as he comes, demands and gets. The trick is to provide enough program support to keep the older chiefs happy. It's a delicate balancing act."

Although they were in substantial agreement about the magnitude and impact of these dowries, lower-echelon administrators offered differing analyses of *why* the dowries were in fact so large. One took the view that it reflected the long-lived nature of a chief's position: "Usually, bringing on a new chief is a lifetime deal. A chief doesn't take his first position until he's usually in his forties, and when he's pushing sixty or so, some ten or fifteen years down the line he isn't likely to take a new position. As a result, all the chiefs recognize that 'when you go there, you get as much as you can.' They all recognize that this is also true for others."

Another, however, came to the same conclusion by quite the opposite logical process. This administrator reasoned that existing chiefs become upset after their dowry is expended, particularly when they see the bulk of the hospital's resources being committed to new chiefs: "This is why chiefs hop around, since they still expect to get their dowry when they come." This administrator continued, "Hop around refers to moving every several years, after their dowry at one institution runs down. Instead of competing for new programs with dowries for new chiefs, the chief will move to another hospital and receive a higher dowry himself."[1] Although this latter administrator recognized that funding strictures could reduce such activity in the future, the basic premise was nonetheless corroborated by the comment, made by another second-echelon administrator, that Oak Memorial had no choice but to match the dowries provided by other hospitals. "There is the market cost of a chief's dowry; we have to compete with what's out there."

The source of both the apoplexy and the resignation noted in second-level administrators was visible when they contrasted what they perceived to be the luxurious character of Oak Memorial's commitment to new chiefs with their own inability to obtain what they believed to be essential personnel and equipment, first for existing chiefs and second (and most frustratingly) for nonclinical support services at the hospital.

With regard to existing chiefs, the second-level administrators were acutely aware of the need for the hospital to satisfy the requests of the service chiefs. In the words of one, "You've got to meet [your chiefs] halfway, more than halfway if possible." Yet a new dowry could make it all but impossible to obtain even the first-priority requests of existing chiefs, since dowries were taken off the top from discretionary capital and personnel funds each year. This frustration was evident in the comments of one mid-level administrator about the recent dowry for the chief of medicine: "There is now little left over in the capital equipment budget after the money for [the chief of medicine] was allocated. We're announcing the capital budget shortly, mounds of documentation will be submitted [to support various requests]. People will think that they will get an equal share like they did last year. People forget from the time that they agreed to [the chief of medicine] coming on board to the time when the funding consequences are clear. Almost a year and a half later, now, the other chiefs forget what they said, and when they can't get the highest priority on their capital-equipment budget, you just can't say 'You can't get it because he's got it.'"

Another second-echelon administrator had a similar reaction to the effect of this same dowry on discretionary operating funds in the hospital's budget: "I found this big hunk of operating budget for the department of medicine. That made me very upset because I didn't get money for a secretary I desperately needed."

This frustration at the degree to which a large dowry consumed available resources was felt even more directly by the nonclinical areas, particularly by support services like housekeeping and dietary. Second-echelon administrators who had responsibilities in these areas believed that personnel and equipment had been so grievously pinched in the past that a critical need existed to redress the balance. One administrator described her situation in particularly direct terms: "If I couldn't have gotten at least one or two bodies in housekeeping, since they were cut back fifteen people the year before, if I couldn't get at least a turnaround, I wouldn't have had any credibility. I understand that fifteen thousand dollar doodads are bought to make people [in the department of medicine] happy and productive, and that's appropriate, because Oak Memorial isn't going to become a premier research hospital on the basis of my housekeeping department."

Another second-level administrator also explained the difficulty of obtaining resources for nonclinical departments in terms of the chief's position within the hospital: "It's very difficult to sit down with a chief of service and say 'let's talk about cutting six positions.' The administration is not strictly managerial in its relationship to the chiefs. However, when you say you havé to cut six positions to a support department head, that head can argue all he wants but either ultimately he'll cut, or he'll have to resign—there's no alternative." The CEO contended, however, that "this year's [significant] cuts as a result of the expenditure cap were largely in the professional [M.D.] areas. Housekeeping, dietary, etc. were essentially untouched. Furthermore, what program cuts were made (such as child psychiatry) were *professional* personnel virtually exclusively."

Another senior administrator confirmed the tension these dowry decisions could create for second-level administrators at Oak Memorial. Summarizing the reaction to the chief of medicine's recent dowry in a distinctly irritated tone, this administrator noted that "when the decision was taken to bring on this new chief, with his harem and his entourage from all over, as well as to assign a lot of equipment and a lot of space to this new service, . . . it was clear to [second-level administrators] that there are in fact some new programs that are not going to be cut at all, even though there are programs that the [second-level administrators] would perhaps prefer to have that will be cut. . . . There was a lot of frustration among them and their department heads and managers as a result of this particular decision. This anger had to be resolved by a lot of one-on-one meetings with them."

Anecdotally capsulizing the perspective second-level administrators took toward the apparent institutional power of the hospital's service chiefs, one of them told a story about the reaction of physicians at another teaching hospital when the intensive care unit (ICU) at that hospital was closed because of lack of adequate nursing staff. Stunned by "what they perceived to be a lapse of authority, you could watch the physicians scatter as they all went running in search of new sources of power. They were used to thinking that power resided in certain places and that they had their access lines to that power, and when their ICU got closed down all their assumptions about institutional power collapsed. As a result, they started writing everybody: letters to their chiefs, to the president of the hospital, they telephoned members of the board, anyone to get that unit operating again."

Overall, then, second-echelon administrators were not nearly as sanguine about the role of service chiefs at Oak Memorial as were the hospital's senior administrators. They felt that revenue constraints were not nearly as important with regard to chiefs' issues and programs as they should be, and these administrators felt that their own jobs were much more difficult as a result. In a very fundamental sense, despite their recognition of the clinical chiefs' importance to the overall mission of the hospital, these administrators tended to feel that the pursuit of prestigious teaching and research programs had some important negative consequences for revenue and for resource allocation.

Service Chiefs' Perspective

In seeking to define the character of interactions between physicians and administrators at Oak Memorial, we readily concluded that the service chiefs acted as proxies for the entire medical staff. Indeed, since chiefs typically were appointed from outside the service itself — selected primarily by a search committee of the medical school, including the hospital's existing chiefs plus the CEO, and since the chiefs themselves were central in recruiting and appointing new faculty and physicians within the service, it was not surprising that for all intents and purposes each chief spoke for his service's medical staff, particularly since he was accountable for their activities.

The relationship between the service chiefs and administrators at Oak Memorial was a complicated one. Although there was broad general support among the chiefs for what they perceived to be the overarching strategic requirements of the hospital as a whole, that support tended to splinter when a given chief found himself denied something he believed essential. The success of this classic "It's a good idea but don't cut my service" response varied along several dimensions, as will be discussed below. Moreover, there often appeared to be substantial divergence between general principles and specific decisions as they affected requests for resources.

PERCEPTIONS OF THE ADMINISTRATION

There was, first, a strong and genuine respect for the integrity and administrative capabilities of the hospital's CEO. Indeed, the chiefs uniformly described him as one of the best hospital administrators in the country. The new chief of medicine called him "the best hospital administrator I have ever seen." Speaking more generally about the quality of Oak Memorial's administration, the chiefs were equally positive. Comments ranged from "they're terrific" to "they are tough but very supportive" to "far more reliable, more honest, more fair, and more aboveboard than other hospital administrators."

Despite these readily offered encomiums, most of Oak Memorial's chiefs also made various comments about the existing administration that appeared to belie this unconditional praise. A common criticism was that the second-echelon administrator assigned to their service was powerless or even devious. One chief said, "For the first years, I fell into the trap by talking to an administrator who was completely powerless and wasted my time." Another noted that although his present administrator is "first rate," "He replaced someone who was awful; he talked around everything, was very smooth but never solved anything." A third, with reference to a difficulty his service was still seeking to solve, commented of the second echelon, "We tried these people first but they didn't come up with anything."

Finally, one chief dismissed the whole notion of Oak Memorial's hierarchically structured administration: "I used to deal with two administrators, now I deal with four. That's absurd. Administrator number four has no authority and administrator number three just sends it up to administrator number two to make the decision or sometimes sends it to administrator number one. I totally fail to see the importance of administrators number three and four with regard to my department." This chief explained his adamancy as based in part on the lack of background and rapid turnover of lower-level administrators: "Level-three and level-four administrators are never around for a great length of time and never understand the nature of the problem within [my service]. Is it really worthwhile to give tutorials to level-three and level-four administrators that may turn over every eighteen months?"

Implicit within this last comment was still another indication that chiefs did not always act in accordance with the administration's formal decision-making system. Rather, they exercised an option that all chiefs except one confessed they had used in the past: to take a problem directly to Oak Memorial's CEO. One chief, for example, commented, "I've been to [the CEO] on a number of occasions" to discuss what he (the chief) perceived to be important matters. Another said, "Oh, I'll talk to the [second-level administrator], but in the end it will go to [the CEO] if there is no adequate resolution." A third qualified his willingness to circumvent channels by saying, "I won't cry wolf unless there's a big wolf there, but for big problems I wouldn't hesitate."

Perhaps the most revealing comment, however, came from a chief who linked going directly to the CEO with what he perceived as the responsibility of senior administrators for the negative responses of the second-echelon administrators. But he also carried the issue beyond meeting with the CEO to marshaling additional support from his fellow chiefs, noting that "from the beginning it was clear that if the administrative personnel didn't meet my demands, it was because [the CEO] wouldn't let them." He continued that if an important request was refused when sent through proper channels, "I would take it up with [the COO] and either agree with him or, if not and it's of paramount importance, I would probably go to [the CEO]. I also would probably go to my other colleagues and try to generate support, since I clearly can't take on [the CEO] alone."

The most consistent theme that ran through the chiefs' interactions with Oak Memorial's administration was the various techniques by which they satisfied their resource needs. It's important, first, to note that no chief felt he was ever making anything other than a reasonable request.

The range of comments, from one chief who said, "I don't ask for the sky, and I don't pad the budget" to a more cynical chief who said, "I ask for the reasonable, and I get the reasonable less 10 percent," was rather consistent in this respect. Moreover, most of Oak Memorial's chiefs felt strongly that meeting their service's requests also was important for the hospital as a whole. One chief's statement that "what's good for my department tends to be good for the hospital" mirrored a sentiment commonly repeated among the chiefs.

As we noted above in the section on middle management, many of the chiefs' requests were in fact routinely met by the normal budgeting process. One second-level administrator, when asked if his chiefs usually expected to receive at least their first capital-equipment priority, unhesitantly responded, "absolutely." There was nevertheless an extrabudget process for both equipment and personnel that took place ad hoc throughout the budget year. Although senior administrators discouraged reliance upon this secondary allocation system, some chiefs found it a useful way to evade the stringencies of the official budget. One chief explained his use of this supplementary process by noting that "programs really do change over the course of a year."

As we indicated previously, however, by far the most significant effect upon the chief's ability to obtain desired resources was caused by dowries. As we will see, this was true both positively — in terms of what a new chief received — and negatively — in terms of what existing chiefs subsequently did not obtain.

THE CHIEFS' VIEW OF DOWRIES

With the exception of the chief of psychiatry, every chief at Oak Memorial had received a dowry when he came to the hospital, but there were several variants on how these arrangements were consummated. The most common was a more or less protracted set of negotiations between a candidate and the CEO, followed by a letter of understanding from the CEO. The most explicit description of this process came from the hospital's recently arrived chief of medicine: "I articulated to [the CEO] what the needs were, in terms of the following: X is the present budget plus an inflation factor, Y is the budget support needed for the department once it's in a new steady state, and Z are the one-time costs needed to put it in a new steady state. That resulted in a one-hour discussion with [the CEO] alone, about X, Y, and Z, which in turn resulted in a letter of commitment from him agreeing with these plans." Another chief summed up the process succinctly when he commented that, in his case, "Most of the power politics took place in the negotiations and very little after that."

A third chief noted of his experience, "when I came here, there was a package of research equipment and space which I really needed. We had nothing written, just a handshake, which I was warned not to do, but it worked out fine."

The reason for the existence of these dowries, in the eyes of the chiefs, was the need to obtain the space, personnel, and equipment necessary for pursuing one's intended programs at a new hospital. As explained by the chief of orthopedic surgery, "These dowries emerged in the response to your ability to get things once you're there. If you don't have it out front you're in trouble; you don't have much leverage after that." Perhaps the most explicit delineation of the logic behind the chief's dowry came, once again, from the newly arrived chief of medicine:

> You're in the best position as a chief to negotiate when you take the job; you're in the second best position when you're prepared to leave it. No matter how good your personal relations are at the hospital, if you can't achieve your personal goals for the department, then you should consider other options. It's something that's unspoken, but this proposition operates in the background. The intelligent thing for the candidate to do is express his needs, not take the assurance of administration [no matter how well motivated] of "we want what you want, we want a strong department, and therefore you have nothing to worry about." It's naive to take that kind of assurance. The person giving you the assurance is under multiple pressures and his tenure may be limited. If a radiologist quits next year, these assurances can be broken because of the need to bring in a new person. It's important to establish a long-range commitment and make it as tight and simple as possible.

The negative side to chiefs' dowries was shown in the comments of some of the longer-sitting chiefs at Oak Memorial. As one dryly summarized the consequences these multimillion-dollar commitments had for the rest of the chiefs, "There is only so much available; therefore something has to give!" Another, just as dryly, agreed that "existing chiefs lose out; I think that's true," and a third, somewhat more combatively, said of his own situation, "After ten years, the honeymoon is over."

A number of chiefs also questioned the wisdom of such enormous one-shot allocations of the hospital's resources. In the words of one support service chief, "I think it's an error in university hospital planning." A second concurred and offered the following comments about his own dowry by way of explanation: "Whatever I asked for they gave me, and I therefore had to take the job. This is idiotic; it's a poor investment policy because every little specialty gets everything, and you get a lot of white elephants. The hospital's development is unbalanced."

There was, in sum, considerable concern among at least some chiefs, even though they themselves had done well when they came, that the dowry process distorted the hospital's overall program development.

OTHER RESOURCE ALLOCATION CRITERIA

These rather general criticisms of the dowry process were supplemented by concerns about a more specific allocation issue, the relative ability of different service chiefs to obtain resources. This encompassed at least three likely areas of conflict: between current dowry obligations to two or more new chiefs; between a dowry obligation and the hospital's annual operating and capital equipment budgets; and between service chiefs for discretionary resources within the hospital's annual budget.

In all the instances above, it appeared that concern with institutional prestige, heavily laced with awareness of the size and the revenue contribution of each service, determined Oak Memorial's resource priorities. At the time of the study, the clearest beneficiary of this approach was the hospital's department of medicine, which satisfied all three essential criteria: it was the largest department in the hospital, had a strong professional reputation, and contributed substantial revenue (according to one chief, medicine usually filled 80 percent of the hospital's beds). This strong structural position, combined with the impact of the new chief of medicine's dowry, reinforced the other service chiefs' sense that they were in competition with medicine for resources.

The conflicts over resources at Oak Memorial were related to both financial support and research space. As the new chief of medicine described it, resource issues "are very concrete in a teaching hospital. They can be calculated in terms of square feet, in terms of dollar support for people, and in terms of dollar support for people's programs." The competitive element in obtaining these resources was apparent to chiefs whose services satisfied some but not all of the three key allocation criteria noted above. Orthopedic surgery, for example, was a new department recently spun off from surgery. It was clearly expected to be a revenue generator,[2] and its research activities were productive and growing. Moreover, the chief had come to Oak Memorial only three years before, and he was still in the process of utilizing his own substantial dowry. Nonetheless, this chief felt that he was in an unequal position from which to compete with medicine for key resources. "My own major difficulty," he commented, "is to obtain new space on a temporary basis until we get into the new lab." Yet he felt that despite his best efforts little additional space had been forthcoming: "I spoke with [the CEO] four or five months ago, I thought we had a commitment from him, but it's still not solved." This chief's analysis of his inability to obtain what he felt he needed — indeed what he perceived as part of his own dowry—turned on the status of the department of medicine within the hospital. He continued: "Let's face it, we're not naive, the department of medicine has tradition, numbers, and the needs of the hospital on its side. Part of our space problem may be that we got caught in the crunch with negotiations with the department of medicine for the new chief."

This perception of the chiefs' relative ability to obtain resources was confirmed by the chief of neurology, another small but well regarded and revenue-generating service. This chief felt that a teaching hospital like Oak Memorial had to recognize a variety of different needs, including academic as well as revenue requirements. He concluded that "there would be one other factor in this discussion: Do certain chiefs have more weight with [the CEO]? The answer is yes. Neurology would be at a disadvantage compared with larger departments. This is not unfair, because if surgery fills two hundred beds and neurology has only twenty-five, it's not the same. Of course there are countervailing influences because we're a very effective department. However, all things being equal, the chief of medicine is more likely to get what he wants than is the chief of neurology."

This interplay among prestige, size, and revenue-generating capacity also appeared to work to the disadvantage of some of Oak Memorial's less well positioned services. One chief noted of academically based arguments to support resource requests, "The higher levels of administration will respond in terms of the standing of the individual chief. For example, 'chief X is really a weak academician and thus to allocate resources to the service would be a poor investment; that chief runs an academically weak service and thus is a waste of money.'" Speaking subsequently of financial requests, this same chief again noted the importance of the service's previous performance: "Success breeds success: we've done well before. Someone else might come in with the same argument but get short shrift. [The CEO] will say, 'so-and-so has approached me and I'm really reluctant; he's not done too well before.'" Summarizing this issue of the comparative return to the different chiefs from Oak Memorial's resource-allocation decisions, the chief cited above concluded that the hospital's CEO "is obligated to allocate his resources as best he can to produce for the hospital."

One very interesting concomitant of this competition among service chiefs was the combined effort of the department of fiscal affairs, the board of trustees, and the hospital's senior administrators to establish a mechanism to put pressure on services that the department of fiscal affairs saw as a financial loss to the hospital. Although a full exploration of this "special projects subcommittee" of the board of trustees will follow in a subsequent section, it is worth noting here that in at least two instances the prestigious character of a service's academic and research program was sufficient to insulate that service fairly well from its revenue failings.

RESOURCE-INFLUENCING TECHNIQUES

Three additional aspects of the service chiefs' ability to obtain resources at Oak Memorial bear mentioning. First, there is the apparent tendency of some physicians to utilize the standards of the national medical education committees as justification for resource requests. One surgical subchief at Oak Memorial described this strategy rather pointedly: "Many individuals here use the liaison committees from Chicago—the LCME and the LCGME [3]—against the medical school itself and hide behind them as if they were concrete pillboxes in a war. They can be powerful levers in the competitive scramble for resources and patients and all too often are used as weapons for individual gain."

There were, in fact, a number of instances when professional standards set by specialty associations were cited as one basis for additional personnel or capital equipment requests. One chief, for example, relied upon the personnel standards set by his specialty association as part of his effort to obtain several new technicians: "I needed an extra technician at a time when the hospital was putting a freeze on personnel. The yardsticks of [the specialty association] showed that two additional technicians were needed, but we were willing to settle for one."

Second, several chiefs believed that, when pressed, the senior administrators had no real choice but to meet their requests. This sense of there being no alternative to compliance was expressed in several different ways. One chief argued this position rather bluntly: "We're a fully salaried department, so I can't imagine it would make much sense for the hospital to deny us what we need. The bottom line at a hospital like Oak Memorial is that it can't afford to say no to its physicians." This chief elaborated by stating that the hospital's administrators could not "afford" to refuse a chief's requests because they were unable to judge the medical importance of the issues at hand: "The problem is that there isn't any nonphysician administrator who can second-guess me. There can't be. Once you get to be a [prestigious medical school] professor, then you know whereof you speak." Extending his argument to administrators who were also trained physicians, this chief concluded that even in this instance, "Outside one's field, it becomes difficult to know what other areas might need."

On a similar but differently focused note, Oak Memorial's new chief of medicine commented that a teaching hospital's administrators really had no alternative but to supply a key chief with the resources he required. Speaking again of the importance of retaining the option to resign, he contended, "If you're doing a good job, as perceived locally and nationally, it's dangerous for the institution to fire you. First of all, it's very expensive. And second of all, it's hard to get someone to replace you if you quit in a huff and announce that the position of chief at the institution in question is not viable."

The third, final aspect of chiefs' interactions with Oak Memorial's administration concerned the "squeaky wheel." In the view of most chiefs there was in fact a relation between being vocal about one's requests and having them met. Some chiefs took a rather analytic view of this. The chief of orthopedic surgery, for example, commented that "talking and pushing is a factor; it's hard to tell how important it is." Similarly, the chief of neurology said, "I think personality and screaming play a larger role than they should."

These rather detached views were confirmed by the more personal situations of several other chiefs at Oak Memorial. One chief of a powerful service who had been at the hospital a number of years mused, "Perhaps I'm missing something along the way that maybe we should be doing that I'm not pushing hard enough for." Another chief commented rather tartly, "In the first five years I didn't complain enough." The CEO put it somewhat more delicately, but equally clearly: "Since some chiefs are more aggressive in personality and other chiefs are more self-effacing, personality may have some impact on our decisions."

The Role of Fiscal Affairs

There is one final element in the decision-making equation at Oak Memorial that played a key role in resource allocation. This was the strong antagonism with which several of the chiefs had come to view the administration's fiscal affairs department. There were two basic sources of this tension. The first was programmatic and reflected certain chiefs' sense that fiscal affairs had not been particularly forthcoming in helping their services with projected new ventures. One chief summed up this perspective with the following comment: "I think it's a brilliant administration, but if there's one flaw, and it's certainly not only my own opinion, it's in the fiscal affairs crowd." This chief noted of his own situation that although "they put no pressures on me at all," fiscal affairs had taken "six months to respond" to a new proposal from his service.

Another chief told of an incident in which he discovered that fiscal affairs had, without his knowledge, called Blue Cross to ascertain whether an existing program in his service met reimbursement criteria. As a result, reimbursement for the program was canceled, and it took considerable effort by the chief's "working level" administrator to arrange for reimbursement to be restored.

The second focus of tension between fiscal affairs and specific chiefs was the work of the special projects subcommittee of the board of trustees. This subcommittee had been formed some five years before to give the finance committee of the board more detailed analyses of fiscal problem areas at the hospital. Although it did report to the finance committee, and despite its having both the hospital's CEO and the COO as ex officio members, the subcommittee appeared to be largely a new, higher-powered operational arm of fiscal affairs. Fiscal affairs, with final approval by top administration, selected all three problem services that the subcommittee studied and also provided its entire staff.

It was thus fiscal affairs that the selected services perceived as originating the decision to undertake a study. The studies reflected substantial disagreement between fiscal affairs, on the one hand, and the chiefs and "working level" administrators on the other as to how indirect costs were to be defined. In the study of psychiatry — the one that generated the most contention — fiscal affairs had initially sought to assign many indirect costs on the basis of the service's square footage. After numerous vociferous protests from psychiatry (a service that had no technical facilities whatever) that it was being assessed charges for the high-technology requirements of other specialties, fiscal affairs agreed to set the indirect cost figure closer to what outside rental space would cost.

Although the special projects subcommittee's other two studies had not provoked a particularly strong reaction — most likely because they generated little if any administrative action — the study of psychiatry caused considerable controversy within the service. As an outgrowth of the study, there had been for several years a monthly meeting between members of the fiscal affairs task force assigned to the psychiatry project and various psychiatry-service physicians and administrative workers. The goal of these meetings in the eyes of fiscal affairs was to find ways to help psychiatry reduce its structural deficit (even when the service performed according to budget, its deficit remained several hundred thousand dollars). In the view of one participant from fiscal affairs, "we focus on marketing, trying to develop programs that will carry through the dips in summer, for example."[4]

This participant did note, however, that the only long-term solution was to reduce the service's high bad debt and free care ratio: "I've stressed that psychiatry has to change its payer mix — it needs more Blue Cross patients who can and will pay their way after their annual Blue Cross psychiatric coverage runs out." Also, in the words of the CEO, "The M.D.s had to stop promising reductions in fees to patients without an objective review by the fiscal office."

From the perspective of the psychiatry service, however, this process did not appear either so rational or so benign. In the words of one psychiatrist who had been involved in these meetings, "I really don't know how costs are assigned to this unit. I've asked fiscal, and asked and asked." The meetings themselves were, in this participant's opinion, distinctly unpleasant: "The tone in the meetings is constantly negative. I leave with a headache." Moreover, psychiatry had a strong sense that the service was substantially at risk. As the chief put it, "Our goal is teaching, training. We have to make sure that accounting and fiscal services don't destroy our reason for being."

Yet despite this high level of concern with fiscal affairs, the chief of psychiatry felt that at present his service and its programs were not in serious danger. In his words, "We've been scrutinized more than other departments, but I don't feel picked on. The hospital realizes what we do; I don't feel any lack of support." It thus appeared that despite these difficulties, the academic aspect of the psychiatry service at Oak Memorial was sufficiently well regarded and well known that, although it could not insulate the service from pressure, it could prevent revenue concerns from interfering with the service's ongoing activities.

Summary

In general, the character of resource-related decision-making at Oak Memorial Medical Center can be summarized in five points:

- The essential behavioral incentives that influenced resource allocation were the lower-echelon administrators' concerns for revenue and the service chiefs' concern for prestige.
- An important set of informal processes influenced the final decisions on resource allocation.
- Dowries had played a major role in the past, and the effects of many existing dowries would continue.
- The role of fiscal affairs was central to a complete and accurate understanding of the resource implications of prestige-related decisions.
- The array of structural and behavioral levers in decision making strongly favored the medical staff; sooner or later Oak Memorial's chiefs of service usually got what they wanted.

CHAPTER 8
An Analysis of the Two Power Equilibria

The case studies in chapters 4–7 provide a real-world laboratory in which to test, develop, and enrich our thesis on the hospital power equilibrium. They also allow us to compare and contrast the characteristics of power equilibria in teaching and community hospitals. Perhaps most important, through their complexity and richness, the cases give us an opportunity to explore the theory's capacity to respond to current cost containment programs and its implications for appropriate changes in their design. In this chapter we begin to assess some of these issues.

Methodological Questions

An important methodological question that lies at the heart of our research concerns the usefulness of conclusions drawn from field research in just two hospitals. Obviously, those who consider only statistically significant comparisons of large data banks to be "scientifically valid" will look askance at conclusions drawn from a sample of two. We strongly believe, however, that although statistically verifiable information has made important contributions to society's understanding of the health sector, quantitative methodology cannot capture the complexity and richness of hospital organization. More important, statistical conclusions are often misleading when the central analytical question shifts from the descriptive "what" to the more difficult — but for policy purposes more essential — analytic "why." Indeed, as we sought to demonstrate in chapter 2, existing analyses of hospital behavior have all but ignored what we believe is the crucial variable — the hospital's structure of decision-making power — precisely because that variable cannot be captured adequately by quantitative methodologies.

In selecting a qualitative or case methodology it is essential to consider the types of conclusions that can validly be drawn from such studies. Clearly it would be foolhardy to suggest that *every* hospital's internal decision-making structure and process will replicate those described in chapters 4 through 7. Indeed, as most hospital researchers realize, there is no such thing as the "typical" American hospital. Every institution has a unique configuration based on its history, location, ownership, medical staff, patient mix, regulatory environment, and so on. Since *all* hospitals are ultimately anomalous, one must be careful about drawing universal conclusions from almost any sample, no matter how large. It is thus important to stress that we are not attempting to generalize about all hospitals. Rather, we believe that some illuminating observations about only a few — even only two — hospitals can suggest highly important conclusions about the appropriateness of existing public policy. If two distinctly different institutions appear to have rather similar internal decision-making structures, which in turn are diametrically different from those presumed by federal and state health policy, then we feel that important inferences about the failure of current cost containment efforts can reasonably be made. Further, such divergence, in the light of other available knowledge, also appears to justify consideration of how public policy might best be restructured to achieve effective cost control in the hospital sector.

In short, we believe that if these cases demonstrate that the hospital power equilibrium thesis can provide a satisfactory political theory of the hospital, and if this political theory is considerably at odds with the conventional wisdom upon which current public policy toward hospitals is based, then our methodology will have proved its value. Moreover, if the observations we present "resonate" with sophisticated observers of the American hospital scene, as we believe they will, then the conclusions we draw are valid considerations in future public policy debates. With all this in mind, we now turn to an analysis of the findings presented in chapters 4 through 7.[1]

Theoretical Implications of the Case Studies

The thesis we put forward in part 1 contained a series of assertions about the structure of power within hospitals and its implications for the seemingly ceaseless intrahospital pressure for institutional growth. In chapter 2 we asserted that resource decisions were made not by the hospitals' formally constituted officials, but through a fluid and complex power struggle; that this power struggle was institutionalized in a de facto equilibrium to preserve organizational survival; that the medical staff generally dominated this institutional power equilibrium, primarily through physicians' control of uncertainty within the hospital's "production" function; that other occupational groups, in particular nurses, were seeking to improve their relative status within the power equilibrium through increased professionalism; and that physician domination of the decision-making process was under constant but thus far ineffective challenge both by administrators and by the hospitals' other occupational groups. In chapter 3 we further asserted that physicians utilized their dominance within the hospital's power equilibrium in accordance with their own behavioral incentives; and that the modus vivendi that enabled the power struggle to remain in equilibrium — and thus to ensure institutional survival — was predicated on satisfying these various behavioral incentives through continual institutional growth.

We believe that our research demonstrates the likely validity of the hospital power equilibrium theory. As table 3 indicates, the research was conducted in two disparate institutions, with contrasting strategic orientations, organizational structures, programmatic processes, and physician motivations. Nevertheless, the case studies also suggest a remarkable commonality of purpose and outcome within these institutions' resource-related decision processes. Indeed, it is precisely this fundamental similarity that indicates that the hospital power equilibrium theory can provide the conceptual basis for constructing more effective cost containment programs. Some of the more significant disparities are discussed below.

ADMINISTRATORS VERSUS PHYSICIANS

When we look at both Peninsula Community and Oak Memorial, it becomes clear that their formally constituted management — the administrators — did not make the key decisions for their institutions. On the contrary, at both institutions, the decision-making process for day-to-day operational as well as strategic policy matters was situated within a power relationship between administrators and physicians: at Peninsula Community, the fundamental axis of authority ran from physicians with the largest practices; at Oak Memorial it ran from the physicians with the greatest research-related professional prestige — the chiefs of service and particularly the new chief of medicine. Although at Peninsula the administrators sought to maximize financial viability, whereas at Oak Memorial they sought to balance both prestige and fiscal concerns, at *neither* site did administration dominate the institution's preeminent physicians. Quite the contrary: the evidence from both case studies clearly indicates that the medical staff, and within it the most powerful physicians in terms of practice or research-tied prestige, dominated their institutions' resource decisions. At Peninsula, as at Oak Memorial, the medical staff generally obtained what it wanted in the way of capital equipment, program expansion, renovations, and personnel. The administrators at both institutions themselves preferred institutional expansion, though they occasionally had somewhat different priorities for growth than did their key physicians. Nonetheless, even where administrators *disagreed* with their senior medical staff, they rarely if ever could refuse to meet physicians' demands. Instead, their sole option was to delay the inevitable. At Peninsula Community, although the administrators practiced a "consistent" pattern of delay on certain physician-initiated proposals, these new endeavors almost always succeeded eventually if they were backed by preeminent physicians (for instance, the telemetry unit and the endoscopy suite). At Oak Memorial, despite the long formal budget process, administrators felt obligated to give each chief his first-priority equipment request and regularly sought

Table 3 Institutional Comparisons

Issue	Oak Memorial	Peninsula
Strategic orientation		
Primary/secondary orientation	Prestige/financial viability	Financial viability/ physicians' practices
Nature of competition	For residents and "interesting patients"	For patients to fill beds; revenues generally
Physicians' primary orientation	Research	Clinical practice
Patient mix	Includes poor (Medicaid, high bad debt)	Relatively well-to-do; few Medicaid
Expansion	Much; new space, new subspecialties; new equipment	Less; mainly equipment and renovation
Organizational design		
CEO's span of control vis-à-vis physicians	Chiefs only	Potentially all physicians
Organizational tiers	Several	Few
Group practice structure	One per specialty	Multiple, leading to competition among groups in same specialty
Physicians' involvement in operating budget	Chiefs highly involved within parameters set by senior management	Relatively little except for hospital-based practice
Program processes		
Capital budget process	Formal, involving several layers of decision making	Informal; no capital budget per se; senior administration makes most decisions
New program requests	Chief is entrepreneur; chief is filter for subchiefs	Any physician can be entrepreneur
New program approval	New programs generally part of dowry	Ad hoc; relies on congruence of financial and practice incentives
Informal physicians' activities	Some "end runs"; to senior administration only	Some "end runs"; to both senior administration and board
Ultimate ploy	Chief resigns	Withdraw patients
Formal activities	Dowry agreements between chief and CEO; chiefs work through formal structure (not committees)	Committee system; CEO approval
Informal administrative activities	Make deals with vociferous physicians; commit to subsequent year	Delay; "we're working on it"
Physician motivation		
Central concerns	Research and publication to attain tenure; respect of peers necessary for future research grants	Practice building; respect of peers necessary for patient referrals
Financial motives	Increased salary, research support (e.g., practice funds)	Personal income
Career track	Becoming a chief	Building a big practice
Chief's tenure	For "life"	Rotating

to pacify those with unsatisfied requests by giving them priority in the following year's budget.

Given the structure of the power equilibrium at both hospitals, it is not surprising that administrators felt uncomfortable giving a flat no to a physician's request. At Peninsula Community, physicians who were key power brokers were acutely aware of their perceived, if never mentioned, potential to withdraw their patients or their practices from the hospital. To recall the chief of surgery's observation, "I suppose that [patient withdrawal] is something, however, that the administrator must think about in the back of his mind." This perception by Peninsula Community's medical staff is not surprising, given their well-utilized ability to embarrass CEOs before the board of trustees, and indeed their success in "facing down" a former administrator.

At Oak Memorial, although the administrator had successfully precluded powerful physicians from making end runs to the board of trustees, the reality of the administrator/physician power structure was much the same as at Peninsula Community. As one Oak Memorial chief put it bluntly, "The bottom line at a hospital like Oak Memorial is that it can't afford to say no to its physicians." Moreover, there was considerable concern that the budgeting process not ignore longtime chiefs, for fear they might respond by resigning. Perhaps the best indication of this is the CEO's assertion that the threat to leave was not "a unit of currency" at Oak Memorial, in contrast with the new chief of medicine's observation that not only was it "dangerous" for the hospital if a chief "quits in a huff" but, more important, that "you're in the best position as a chief to negotiate when you take the job; you're in the second-best position when you're prepared to leave it."

At both the community and the teaching hospital, then, the fundamental relationship between physicians and administrators remained the same. Although physicians' leverage was constructed around practice withdrawal at Peninsula and prestige withdrawal at Oak Memorial, the perceived power of these threats was essentially equal. The fact that at both institutions these threats were unspoken and, moreover, never actually employed further indicates their parallel function as a key device by which physicians maintained their dominant position within their power equilibria. The threat to withdraw from the institution, like most threats, has power only as long as it is not expressed overtly or presented as an ultimatum. Such implicit threats are among the classic weapons of political conflict, and their presence in the two hospitals studied lends credence to the hospital power equilibrium argument.

Physicians' dominance within the two hospitals can be observed in a variety of other examples mentioned in the case studies. At Peninsula Community, the ease with which attending physicians were able to negate the efficacy of the utilization review program suggests an apparent weakness of the administrators, inasmuch as Peninsula's average length of stay had been criticized by state regulatory authorities as excessive. Similarly, the absence of a formal capital budget at Peninsula Community suggests that the CEO did not wish to confront the medical staff with his capital investment decisions, knowing it would be difficult to make his decisions stick if he made them all known in one document. The ability of affected physicians to hold hostage a new program such as the emergency room until it was designed to include strong protection for their private practices is yet another indication of the inability of Peninsula's administration to override the medical staff.

One can point to a series of similar though differently configured circumstances at Oak Memorial. The intrahospital consequences of offering multimillion-dollar dowries to new chiefs gives an important sense of the chiefs' negotiating power vis-à-vis the administration. In the instance of the dowry for the new chief of medicine, the CEO felt all but required to offer the requested dowry in order to attract the prestige-enhancing chief, despite the frustration he knew would ensue when other chiefs did not receive their top-priority requests for that year. The perceived role of second-echelon administrators as facilitators for their respective chiefs, rather than filters for the institution's overall budget, also suggests that administrators do not feel they are on an equal power plane with the hospital's chiefs of service. Finally, the ability of chiefs to develop large discretionary practice-based funds, and to employ these funds in ways that could expand the hospital's long-term commitments, indicates that administrators feel unable to enforce official budget restrictions on physician-initiated growth.

PHYSICIANS' MOTIVATION

The case studies further suggest that the fundamental behavioral basis upon which physicians reach decisions is quite different in teaching hospitals than in community hospitals, yet it has rather similar consequences for the overall decision process in both types of institution. We found, for example, that physicians at Peninsula Community Hospital grounded their clinical and policy decisions on criteria that reflected a concern for building their medical practices. As such, the relative power of different physicians, as perceived both by the physicians themselves and by administrators, reflected the health and size of their practices.[2] At Oak Memorial, although the fundamental power currency of physicians also included professional reputation among their medical colleagues, the content of this prestige was based on research rather than on practice.

There was, of course, a difference in the orientation of the two hospitals' administrators regarding the form of their physicians' professional prestige. At the teaching institution, the administrators closely shared the medical staff's concept of prestige, whereas at the community hospital the type of prestige that motivated its physicians was not shared in any obvious manner by the administrator. One indication of the extent to which prestige based on research was a shared value for both physicians and administrators at Oak Memorial was the comment of a second-echelon administrator, acknowledging the lesser importance of requests for personnel: "I understand that fifteen thousand dollar doodads are bought to make people [in the department of medicine] happy and productive, and that's appropriate, because Oak Memorial isn't going to become a premier research hospital on the basis of my housekeeping department."

The extent to which research-based and practice-based professional prestige differ was delineated by the relationship within Oak Memorial of its own part-time fee for service physicians with the rest of the full-time salaried medical staff. In the words of one part-time physician: "Even though part-timers fill beds, they have little power in a teaching hospital. In community hospitals, physicians who fill beds have tremendous prestige because they do fill beds."

OTHER OCCUPATIONAL GROUP STRATEGIES

Beyond demonstrating the existence and character of these two hospitals' power equilibria, the case studies also verify the theoretical expectation raised in chapter 2 about the role of the hospitals' other occupational groups. In particular, nursing at Oak Memorial, and to a lesser degree at Peninsula Community, appears to be relying strongly upon a permanent strategy of increased professionalization to secure higher status within the hospital. At Oak Memorial nurses took the position that physicians were "new" to the "collaboration" with them and must be taught to consider nurses as "colleagues." The nurses also adopted patient education as the vehicle for improving their own position vis-à-vis physicians. That in a relatively liberal urban teaching hospital nurses' first strategic step consisted of "confronting physicians directly" if a physician "exhibits unacceptable behavior" suggests how far the present physician/nurse relationship is from anything approaching equality of power. Indeed, the view of one junior physician who interpreted this strategy as "nurses wanting to be doctors" confirms both the distance that lies between these two groups and the threat that physicians perceive from nursing's increasing professionalization.

At Peninsula Community nursing had even less status in the eyes of physicians than it did at Oak Memorial. Instead of building nurses' sense of professionalism through confrontation with physicians, the nursing administrator at Peninsula Community had settled upon a strategy of gaining salary increases for nurses, in part to pave the way for more amicable physician/nurse relations.

Moreover, at Peninsula Community one could clearly see that physicians felt threatened by encroachment from medical professionals other than nurses. They refused to discuss their lab orders with pathology technicians and were comfortable considering alternative tests only with another physician, the pathologist. Additionally, Peninsula Community's obstetricians felt directly threatened by the potential presence in the hospital of midwives, and the private psychiatrists most demonstrably did not appreciate the notion of psychologists and psychiatric social workers staffing the new outpatient clinic.

In sum, the argument in chapter 2 that the hospital is a "seedbed of professionalization," generating persistent yet thus far unsuccessful challenges to physicians' dominant role in decision making appears to be well substantiated by the two case studies.

STRATEGIES BETWEEN PHYSICIANS

The two cases also suggest the extent to which physicians maneuver among themselves to continue or extend their power. At Oak Memorial, for instance, the various chiefs regularly supported or confronted the demands of fellow chiefs, depending on the circumstances. For instance, the chief of radiology and the chief of orthopedic surgery supported each other in their respective requests for a portable fluoroscope and for renovations. Yet the chief of a smaller service felt that his dowry had not been fully realized because it conflicted with that promised to the newer chief of medicine, a perception the chief of neurology reinforced with his observation that "all things being equal, the chief of medicine is more likely to get what he wants than is the chief of neurology." Moreover, a similar set of activities could be observed inside various clinical services. Whereas chiefs tried to maintain their "flexibility" in dealing with subordinate physicians within their departments, subchiefs continued to search for ways to increase their leverage over their chiefs. One subchief sought budgetary control over his subdepartment, while another felt his only tool was to complain regularly. A third subchief responded by adjusting his strategy and concentrating on what he perceived to be an unchallengeable direction, basic research. Finally, there were also clear power breaks—with the accompanying jockeying for position—between full-time salaried physicians and part-time fee for service physicians (as noted above) and between attending physicians and house staff.[3]

There was a parallel although less richly detailed history of internecine warfare at Peninsula Community. There were clear instances of intradepartmental disputes over patient referrals. In the department of medicine, the competition between two separate group practices was so heated that a new consultant had to decide which of the two groups to "join." At the service level, there was a long-term battle between obstetrics and anesthesiology over the lack of epidural anesthesia or twenty-four-hour coverage. There also was a less heated but nonetheless direct confrontation between radiology and pathology over which service would receive its most recent request. Finally, there was a residual issue between the fee for service physicians that dominated Peninsula Community's medical staff and the hospital-based physicians, in which the former tended to disparage the needs of the hospital-based physicians because the latter were not supporting a practice.

INSTITUTIONAL GROWTH INCENTIVES

The two case studies appear to support the major contention of chapter 3, that the permanent group strategies of physicians, administrators, and the hospital's other occupational groups could best be satisfied by continued institutional growth. At both Oak Memorial and Peninsula Community, the fundamental pressure from the medical staff was for new programs, equipment, and space. Moreover, the response of administrators at both institutions was to satisfy these expansionary demands to the greatest extent possible. That the two administrators sought to deflect unfulfilled requests by different strategies takes little away from the common character of the endeavor. Neither does the observation that the behaviors through which the physicians at the two hospitals sought these changes involved different formulations of professional prestige. The outcome clearly remained the same: at the time of the study, both institutions were involved in as much expansion as they could financially digest.

DIFFERENCES BETWEEN THE INSTITUTIONS

The two case studies also suggest that the composition of different hospitals' power equilibria may not vary as greatly as theorized in chapter 2. One of the more surprising results, as we noted before, is that while specific topics and tactical mechanisms differed between the community hospital and the teaching hospital, the outcome was much the same. This similarity of the general power equilibrium structure is even more surprising given the considerable differences in management style between the chief administrator at Oak Memorial and his counterpart at Peninsula Community. One might, for instance, contrast the statements of genuine respect for the CEO from Oak Memorial's chiefs with the sense of Peninsula Community's physicians that their administrator would soon disappear, leaving them to deal with the consequences. One might contrast the formal, overt capital budgeting process, including all chiefs' requests save dowry commitments, at Oak Memorial with the complete absence of a capital equipment budget at Peninsula Community. One might also consider that the ultimate physician end run at Oak Memorial was to the CEO, whereas at Peninsula Community it was behind the CEO's back to the board of trustees.

Despite these dissimilarities, the structure of power remained essentially the same in both hospitals. The senior medical staff, whether the chiefs of the larger services or the attending physicians with the most active practices, almost always got what they wanted. In fact, the strongest administrative sanction at either institution was to delay a request until the following year or perhaps to force the physician to arrange outside funding. In what is perhaps the most telling indicator of the relative strength of physicians and administrators within these two hospitals, the administration rarely if ever uttered the word no.

There is always the possibility, as we said earlier in the chapter, that the two institutions studied were sufficiently atypical to skew the results of our research. While we do not entirely discount that possibility, the structural imbalance between physicians, on the one hand, and administrators, nurses, and other hospital occupational groups, on the other, appears to be so great that only heroic efforts could reequilibrate it. Indeed, the evidence from both this study and prior research is powerful enough to suggest that physicians' hegemony lies at the very core of the present form of American hospital organization.

Cost Containment Issues

The similarities and differences discussed above raise important although often unacknowledged cost containment issues. In particular, the character of the two hospitals' decision-making power equilibria, and the comparative behavior of senior physicians in influencing resource allocation, suggests that existing hospital management control systems are not effective and that current cost containment programs are woefully inadequate. In this section we will explore the broad rationale behind our observations about the two hospitals studied and assess how these observations relate to the structural aspects of existing cost containment policies.

We have grouped our discussion of important policy variables into four general categories: dowries, program development, capital budgeting, and revenue and cost considerations.

THE ROLE OF DOWRIES

As the Oak Memorial case study demonstrates, in a teaching hospital a dowry is considered an essential recruiting tool. In general, dowries provide one-time allocations — for program development, space, equipment — rather than covering ongoing operating costs, although consideration can be given to these latter costs as well. Beyond being a recruitment device, however, dowries reflect the intense competition for prestige among teaching hospitals and their desire to be on the cutting edge of new developments in medicine. For most teaching hospitals the goal is not just to practice but to create state of the art clinical care, since it is upon this that an academic hospital's reputation is based.

The distinction between developing and practicing state of the art medicine in turn helps explain a chief's need to receive a dowry. In the first place, developing state of the art medicine is a research activity, and a dowry provides not only the necessary research facilities, but a suitable platform from which to apply for outside research grants. Moreover, the interrelatedness of medical specialties for both research and teaching militates against allowing "weakness" to appear in any aspect of the hospital's activities. Without strong departments of cardiology and gastroenterology, for example, Oak Memorial would not be able to engage in research related to these subspecialties, nor would it be able to sustain top-quality residencies in medicine or even surgery.[4]

Second, one must consider the role of dowries in allowing physicians to practice state of the art medicine. Here the issue is less clear, since research equipment often has little if any clinical function. Nonetheless, Oak Memorial's newly appointed gastroenterologists and cardiologists can be expected to see at least some patients and to use newly developed procedures in these patients' care. Additionally, these subchiefs can be expected to train residents in new procedures. We can also expect to find aspects of the chief of pathology's new laboratories, which were in his dowry, being used for both clinical care and teaching as well as research. One would anticipate a similar situation in another technology-intensive hospital-based service, radiology. Similarly, although physicians at Peninsula Community did not receive dowries as such, many of their requests were in fact for equipment that would allow them to practice — though not develop — state of the art medicine.

A third issue concerns the implications academic dowries hold for the overall structure of the United States health care system. Because dowries are driven by individual hospitals' recruitment requirements, their institutional financial implications frequently are large, in terms of both their initial investment and their "ripple effect" on operating budgets. Dowries also can distort institutional program planning. Specifically, if a chief resigns a replacement must be recruited, and the dowry required to entice a new chief may divert the hospital's resources to the new chief's research priorities rather than to the overall strategic priorities of the institution. Most important, though, every dowry comes with a substantial social price tag. That is, owing to their idiosyncratic genesis, dowries can lead to unnecessarily expensive and duplicative programs and facilities within the health care system as a whole.

A final issue concerns the likely intrainstitutional consequences of dowries in a period of constrained resources. Until now, hospitals' continued ability to grow has softened the impact of large dowries upon the availability of support for other activities and programs. With the onset of increasingly severe resource constraints in the 1980s, however, administrators in teaching hospitals will face ever more difficult decisions about resource allocation. At Oak Memorial, for example, the senior administrators had considerable trouble buffering the internal institutional reaction to the multimillion-dollar dowry provided to the chief of medicine. It seems safe to say that in the future such conflicts will become increasingly common and increasingly difficult to resolve.

THE PROGRAM DEVELOPMENT PROCESS

Although dowries, program development, and capital budgeting are closely related, program development has several unique features that require separate consideration. For discussion, a "program" will be considered to refer to both clinical services and capital equipment. As such, a "new program" could include one or more of the following: a new medical service not previously offered; the expansion of an existing service; the purchase of new or occasionally replacement equipment; renovations to existing physical structures; construction of entirely new physical facilities.

As figure 3 suggests, a program can be viewed as lying at the intersection of four key actors in the health system: the public sector (including insurers), patients, physicians, and hospital administrators. In some states legislation requires that new program requests undergo a public "determination of need" process, in which a public sector agency reviews hospital plans and must give official approval to programs above a certain size; in other states public sector review is not required. Once in place, the new hospital program usually is paid for in large part by the third-party insurers whose subscribers receive care in that particular institution. Whether public sector input regarding new programs is active, as in "certificate of need" states, or passive, as in those states that choose not to impose specific controls, the policy role of the public sector remains essentially the same. By allowing a new program to be put into place, the public sector agrees with the hospital's premise that the program can satisfy certain patient needs, and it further indicates that it is willing to pay both the hospital and its physicians to treat those needs over an indefinite period.

The case studies suggest that within the hospital new programs undergo a complex process of gestation, formulation, and implementa-

Figure 3 Programs and Health System Actors

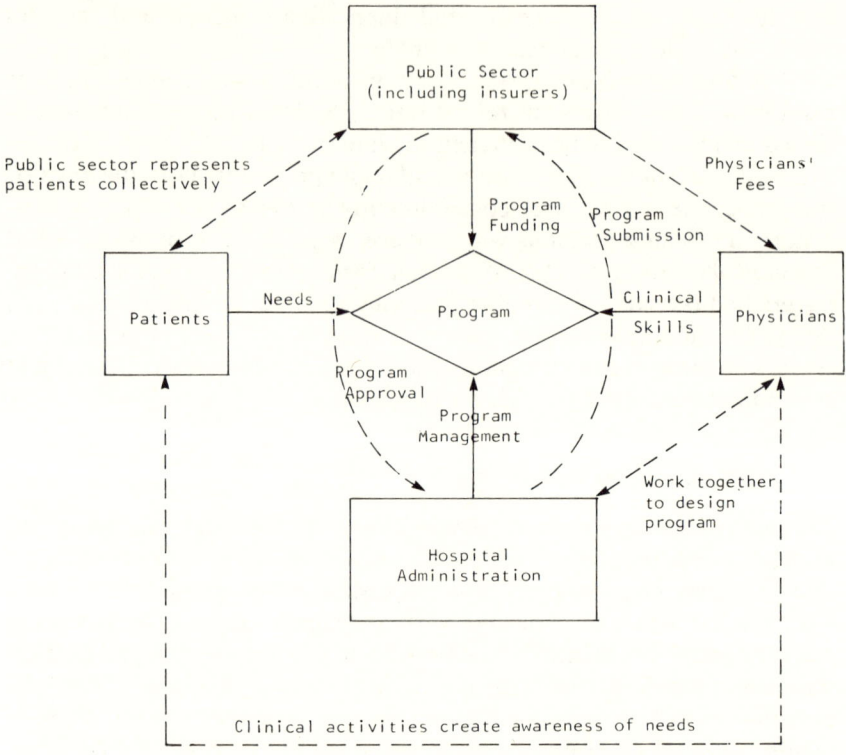

tion. Figure 3 conveys the interactive character of this process. In the state where we conducted our study, these activities were carried out in a laissez-faire fashion rather than through active or directive public mechanisms such as requests for proposals. New program endeavors were generated by a hospital's physicians (occasionally by its administrators), based on their perception of the clinical needs of actual or potential patients. The new programs were then fleshed out through the joint efforts of physicians and administrators and, if they exceeded the certificate of need dollar floor, were submitted for approval. These proposals generally were approved by the state regulatory agency.[5]

At Oak Memorial, a substantial amount of program development was carried out in conjunction with dowry commitments, and even those developments initiated outside the dowry framework had an underlying rationale similar to that for dowries. In both instances, new programs were generated by Oak Memorial's chiefs of service, either jointly, when sitting as the search committee for new chiefs, or independently, when sending up nondowry requests through the hospital's second-echelon administrators.

Although Oak Memorial's senior administrators tried to restrain requests from either format that did not fit their predetermined institutional development strategy, the administrators often shared the chiefs' prestige-based criteria for new programs, and unless there were severe adverse reimbursement implications, they generally appeared to accept demands whether tied to dowries or not.

At Peninsula Community, since there were no dowries as such, new program development was carried out rather more idiosyncratically. Moreover, the underlying rationale for program development appeared to be somewhat different than at Oak Memorial, a divergence we suspect might hold generally between teaching and community hospitals.

As suggested by table 4, program development at Peninsula Community appeared to result from the confluence of physicians' motivation and hospital finances. The source of the idea for the new program always came from an interested physician and always reflected a perceived personal advantage. In some instances the initiating physician wanted the new program in order to practice state of the art medicine, as with the body scanner and the telemetry unit. In other instances the particular physician sponsor believed the new program was important for the development of his or her private practice, as with sports medicine and the endoscopy suite. Finally, some new programs were proposed primarily because they expanded the department's repertoire of clinical services, such as the outpatient psychiatry clinic and the midwife program. Clearly these categories overlap somewhat. The body scanner, for instance, enhanced the private practice of the chief of radiology and expanded the radiology department's available services as well. The three-way classification above simply illustrates that the initial force behind particular programs may be quite different even though the ultimate rationale behind each proposal is to develop the medical practice of the proposing physician.

Of equal importance to physicians' motivations is the second dimension of table 4, in that it suggests why some programs were implemented rather rapidly by Peninsula Community's administration and others were not. The evidence in our case studies clearly suggests that programs likely to be financially beneficial to the hospital were rapidly put in place, while programs that were of no financial benefit or were financially detrimental moved more slowly—although, as noted in the previous section, no program was ever directly disapproved.

In many respects this outcome is precisely what one might expect given the structural cross-pressures on Peninsula Community's administrators. Although the hospital's financial posture required that it grow only in fiscally reimbursable directions, the medical staff's overwhelming influence within its power equilibrium precluded administrators from ever directly refusing to fulfill the physicians' demands. In these circumstances,

Table 4 Reasons for Program Development at Peninsula Community Hospital

Physicians' Motivations for Program Development	Effect on Hospital's Finances	
	Financially Beneficial	No Benefit or Financially Detrimental
Practice of state of the art medicine	Body scanner	Telemetry unit
Primarily reasons of professional practice	Sports medicine	Endoscopy suite
Primarily clinical service expansion	Outpatient psychiatry clinic	Midwife program

one can argue that Peninsula Community's chief administrator had responded as best he could by delaying programs that had substantial support from physicians but were not financially beneficial. This program development pattern at Peninsula does suggest, however, that one central health policy question is whether it is in society's best interests to have new programs initiated largely by physicians based on their individual practice requirements, and filtered by hospital administrators based on the short-run effects on the hospital's financial statement. We will return to this question in the last section of the chapter.

THE CAPITAL BUDGETING PROCESS

In light of the financial concerns just mentioned, the sharp contrast in capital budgeting between the two institutions appears to reflect more than simply chance or managerial style. As the case studies spelled out in some detail, the official capital budgeting process at Oak Memorial (beyond dowry decisions) was formal and highly routinized, whereas that at Peninsula Community was informal and ad hoc. However, these contrasting methods of capital budgeting fit quite well with the primary and secondary strategic orientations highlighted in table 3.

Our case study of Oak Memorial clearly suggests that prestige concerns dominated input into the program development process from both physicians and administrators. Moreover, a sizable proportion of these prestige-driven commitments devolved from the dowries given to new chiefs upon their appointment. As a direct consequence of the way Oak Memorial's capital budgeting process was tied to prestige and dowries, that process could — indeed, must — be overt and formal. The administration's principal challenge each year was to meet the cost of newly awarded dowries, to appease other new chiefs whose dowry commitments could not be met that year, and still somehow to satisfy those less recent chiefs who had major new requests that existing dowry commitments precluded. A formal capital budgeting process was therefore essential to assure a new chief that his dowry commitment would be met, either in this budget year or in the following one. Moreover, since all dowry commitments were given with the concurrence of the other sitting chiefs and with their full knowledge of the dowry's content, a formal capital budget not only helped to avoid enormous animosity among physicians, but reminded the sitting chiefs each year why their own major programs might not yet have been funded. In essence, the prestige-and dowry-based character of Oak Memorial's capital budget enabled senior administrators to use the budget formulation process as a mechanism (albeit slight) for managing physicians.

At Peninsula Community, by contrast, the administration's primary strategic orientation was toward financial viability. The character of the medical staff's interest in the capital budget process was not a shared concern, as with institutional prestige at Oak Memorial, but rather reflected a concern with the continued viability of their private medical practices. Further, Peninsula Community did not require recruitment dowries, hence there was no broad physician-accepted basis upon which the administrators could construct an annual capital budget. Quite the contrary, in each budget year, every capital commitment to a particular physician directly reduced the possibility of a capital commitment to every other physician. Worse, the financial viability criterion upon which these decisions were made opened the administration to charges of philistinism from physicians who were left out. Lacking the coordinating effect of chief-controlled clinical departments, faced with proposals based on private practice rather than overall institutional prestige, and confronted with the harsher nature of physicians' dominance within the hospital's power equilibrium (in which previous administrators had been "faced down with fixed bayonets"), Peninsula's senior administrators apparently felt that to institute an official capital budgeting process would unlock a Pandora's box of undesirable responses from physicians. In short, a formal capital budgeting process might become a vehicle physicians could employ to push through financially marginal projects.

It is interesting to note the dual use of Crozier's contention that power flows from maximizing other occupational groups' uncertainty that one will perform one's designated function. Peninsula Community's physicians cloaked every new program request in the language of quality care and increased patient satisfaction, with the implied threat that too little of either could lead to practice withdrawal. Its administrators, retaliating in kind, maintained an ad hoc capital budget that minimized physicians certainty about which proposals, from which physicians, would be approved or about when approval would occur.

It is unlikely that every nonprofit community hospital will have an unstructured and strictly informal capital budgeting process like that observed at Peninsula. For institutions with differently composed occupational groups, different external environments, and differently structured power equilibria, a different method of budgeting may of course exist. This is precisely the type of factor that will vary from institution to institution depending on the character of the power equilibrium. What is significant from a managerial perspective, however, is that the capital budgeting processes observed at Oak Memorial and Peninsula Community fit well with each institution's structural character, power equilibrium, and strategic orientation.

Two important related public policy points arise out of this discussion of program development and capital budgeting. First, at both Oak Memorial and Peninsula Community we found physicians who emphasized that, since their departments were "revenue generators," their capital requests should be approved almost automatically. Since current health policy pressures hospitals to increase revenue, certain physicians can successfully compete for resources on the basis of their ability to do this. Such behavior coincides well with individual hospitals' financial objectives but may not reflect the overall health needs of a hospital's patient population. As such, there may be a lack of congruence between public policy goals and the goals of individual hospitals.

The second public policy issue concerns the relation between capital expenditures and operating costs. Research has indicated that the capital cost of a particular endeavor — be it a program, a building, or a piece of equipment — is only the tip of the cost iceberg.[6] As the case studies suggest, however, this is not a one-time unidirectional relation between a capital expenditure and its associated operating costs. Rather, as shown in figure 4, there is a much more complex set of interrelated activities. Capital costs also create a need for related capital costs and can lead to teaching programs or research endeavors, both of which have capital and operating costs of their own. The kidney transplant service at Oak Memorial is a good example of this, in which a kidney transplant program motivated by institutional prestige required a new dialysis unit, which in turn had its own capital needs. One could speculate that the next step in this development process might be a residency program in nephrology. Thus each capital, operating, research, or teaching requirement can spawn further requirements in an upward spiral of growth and expansion.

REVENUE AND COST CONSIDERATIONS

The concern for revenues and costs at both Oak Memorial and Peninsula Community mirrors the incentives that now exist throughout the United States health delivery system. Looking at the importance of revenue issues

Figure 4 The Vicious Cycle of Capital Costs

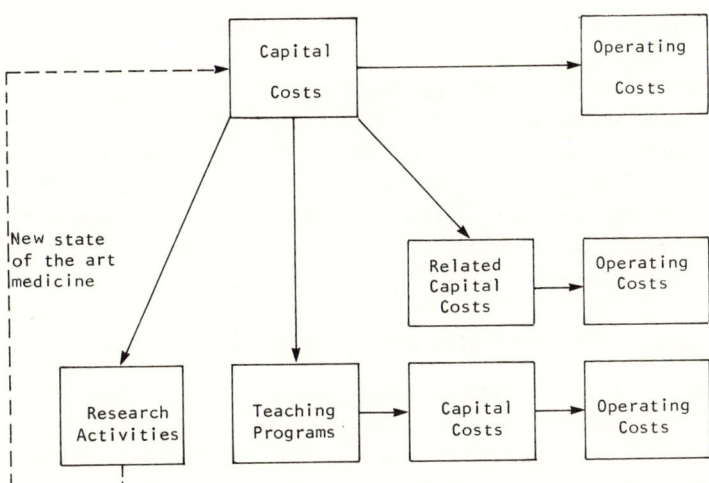

for Peninsula Community, one can readily conclude that there is intense competition for well-insured patients among this state's community hospitals and among community hospitals in general. The increasing fiscal pressure at Oak Memorial suggests that revenue concerns have intruded upon decisions tied to institutional prestige at teaching institutions as well.

This increasingly revenue-dependent situation at Peninsula Community has redirected institutional strategy away from patient needs and aligned it more closely with a strictly corporate competitive market approach. It appears that a similar situation may be evolving at Oak Memorial. The emerging outline of this strategy at Peninsula Community is most clearly visible at the level of program planning, where it has resulted in efforts conceived almost exclusively to improve the hospital's competitive edge. The sports medicine program — which for all intents and purposes is a marketing endeavor — is the most obvious example, though one could also include the outpatient psychiatry clinic because of its importance for the growing — and profitable — occupational health program.

In addition to this increasing attention to revenue, both institutions showed concern about costs. At Oak Memorial there was a growing preoccupation with departments that were "losers," that is, whose costs fiscal affairs believed were greater than their revenues. The outpatient department and psychiatry were considered the two principal culprits.[7] However, we observed no similar concern about reducing costs in departments that were not designated "losers," which is curious, since an excess of revenue over costs is no guarantee of an absence of "fat."

Only minimal attention was paid to costs at Peninsula Community, particularly by physicians. Utilization review was of relatively little consequence. Concern about a particular patient's length of stay, in fact, usually surfaced only when the hospital was full and a physician could not admit a patient.[8] Pressure then arose from the medical staff to discharge the least sick patients. That administrators did not actively seek improvements in the hospital's high length-of-stay profile, despite state regulatory pressure, reflects in part their lack of leverage over physicians' clinical decisions and in part the potentially adverse consequences that shorter lengths of stay, coupled with increasing competition for patients, might have on the hospital's financial picture.

Implications for Health Policy and Management

The issues discussed in this chapter clearly have major ramifications for both institutional management and health policy. First, it seems clear that the United States health care system — at least the nonprofit hospital sector — is highly competitive, but competitive in very specific and, to some degree, socially dubious ways. Teaching hospitals appear to feel substantial pressure to compete for prestige, while community hospitals compete for patients. Unfortunately, in neither situation is there competition to meet the health needs of a given patient population in a cost effective manner. Indeed, the driving force — the dominant competitive pressure — at Oak Memorial and other academic medical centers is to create new state of the art curative medicine. In the case of Peninsula Community and other community hospitals, the competition is to generate more revenue from patients. The appropriateness of the increased utilization and concomitant higher costs created by this competitive environment is one of the most significant health policy questions the country faces. Moreover, it is not at all clear that currently proposed cost sharing mechanisms or other demand-reducing schemes can ameliorate this physician-controlled, utilization-intensive scenario.

Second, the present form of utilization-intensive competition has major resource implications. The quest for institutional prestige has led teaching hospitals to provide enormous dowries to incoming chiefs of service, and these dowries have fueled an expansion of programs, space, and equipment. Competition for patients in community hospitals has led to new programs that provide additional services to those with the "proper" insurance coverage. In both instances the long-run result appears to be distinctly higher overall health care costs. Whether, for example, the patients in Peninsula Community's catchment area need a sports medicine program, or whether patients elsewhere need any of a variety of similar programs being developed by community hospitals competing for patients, pales in significance beside the fact that societal choices with major long-term resource implications are being made by individual physicians and hospitals with only passive — generally reactive — involvement by the society that must pay for those choices.

Third, the complex interrelation between operating and capital budgets has critical consequences for effective cost containment in the future. These budgets — which reflect patient treatment patterns and institutional policy decisions — feed each other in an interactive fashion. Capital growth generates a host of associated operating costs: new machines require new personnel to run them; new intensive care and coronary care units require additional specially trained nurses; and so on. However, it is also important to recognize — as physicians obviously do — that the reverse relation also holds. By generating an overfull operating room schedule, surgeons can create pressure to build additional operating room space; by tying up the operating room with endoscopic procedures, as took place at Peninsula Community, they can make a case for a new endoscopy room. Moreover, physicians almost instinctively generate an infinite number of devices for obtaining new programs, services, facilities, and personnel. They may employ a donated piece of equipment as a lever to demand dedicated space or use the existence of one program to argue for another. At academic hospitals, chiefs may use research funds to add new medical and nonmedical staff to their departments, anticipating that when funding expires the hospital will find itself obligated to continue paying the new salaries. In effect, physicians mix and match their control over operating and capital budgets as necessary to obtain whatever type of growth and technology they happen to desire at the moment.

Fourth, as funds for health care become increasingly limited, the present role of dowries in teaching hospitals may have to change. Incoming chiefs may have to accept less, and new forms of recruitment inducements may have to be developed. Prestige concerns may have to be transmuted into forms of medical activity that are less resource intensive. Further, there are important planning questions concerning regionalization of facilities, programs, and research endeavors that must be addressed. Every hospital may not need state of the art equipment and facilities, and in any event the state of the art probably can be more reasonably priced.

Fifth, the whole question of program development in hospitals must be reconsidered, and a serious reevaluation must be made of the proper role of the public sector in the process. The options include remaining relatively passive, as many states are doing at present; becoming somewhat more involved but awaiting proposals from hospitals and other facilities that might then be evaluated and approved; or becoming intensely active, soliciting programs through requests for proposals from hospitals and other groups.

Finally, and most important of all, new mechanisms must be found to manage provider behavior. Rather than focusing cost containment efforts on the relatively impotent patient, as cost sharing suggests, or on hospitals as though they were unified hierarchical entities, as regulation has attempted to do in the past, states, third-party insurers, and the federal government must begin to take a more active role in managing the activities of the two key decision-making provider groups: physicians and administrators.

We believe that more direct management of key hospital decision makers — particularly physicians — has become essential if the health care system is to guarantee all citizens adequate access to quality care at reasonable cost. At present, socially critical decisions about the types of health care needed and their delivery sites are being made on an unplanned, ad hoc basis by the very physicians and administrators who gain by channeling them into institutionally supportive directions. What is required to counteract these forces are new and distinctly different forms of regulation — regulatory approaches that are both more comprehensive and targeted more accurately on key health delivery actors than those that now exist. In part 3 we outline some proposals for the structure of these new approaches.

PART 3
Cost Containment, Public Policy, and the Hospital Power Equilibrium

We concluded part 2 with a series of questions about the ways United States health care resources will be allocated in the future. In this part we build on that discussion to propose a variety of changes to existing hospital regulatory systems, principally those concerned with reimbursing hospitals and physicians for the services they provide.

This last part of the book is premised on our belief that a hospital and physician reimbursement system is, both conceptually and practically, a management control system. Properly designed, a reimbursement system should ensure the effective and efficient use of the resources society devotes to health care delivery in hospitals. As such, the system can be analyzed, critiqued, and redesigned as necessary by relying on the fundamental principles of management control system theory.

In the context of this analytic framework, two related points constitute the thrust of part 3. First, management control systems inside individual hospitals must be restructured to include physicians as well as administrators in the management control process. Second, more highly centralized state-level systems need to be designed (redesigned in the case of existing centralized systems) to incorporate relevant concepts from management control theory as it has been developed in the corporate sector, particularly for multidivisional corporations. Only by introducing more sophisticated and effective management control systems, properly designed to meet the characteristics of both individual hospitals and the several health care "markets" in which they operate, can we successfully contain health care expenditures without jeopardizing patients' access to quality care.

CHAPTER 9
The Need for Centralized Management Control Systems

In chapter 1 we outlined the conceptual limits of the present debate between increased reliance on market forces (particularly through the mechanism of patient cost-sharing) as contrasted with strengthened state and federal regulation. We argued that neither alternative, as framed at present, can satisfactorily respond to the unique multiple-actor structure of the health care "industry." We then suggested that each hospital's internal decision-making structure reflects a complex power equilibrium that will confound competitive approaches and existing regulatory systems alike.

The competitive/cost sharing approach presumes that patients, through their decisions to purchase insurance and seek care, can exercise appropriate control over the health care system. Consequently, cost sharing proponents advocate dismantling existing state-level efforts to control hospital activities, arguing that increased out-of-pocket payments will lead patients to reduce their overall demand for care and to insist that their physician-agents use fewer hospital resources in treating them. In this market-based model, external economic pressure based on patients' purchasing decisions will suffice to bring unnecessary or excessive hospital expenditures into line.

Although we discussed the likely equity, health status, and financial implications of cost sharing in chapter 1, we have not as yet examined the behavioral assumptions inherent in most cost sharing proposals. It may be helpful, therefore, to begin this chapter with a brief analysis of the structural limitations of these proposals.

Cost Sharing and Hospital-Based Programs

As parts 1 and 2 have indicated, there are major incentives for institutional growth in the present health care system, incentives that are deeply rooted in the values of the system's principal decision makers — physicians and administrators. Physicians who practice in teaching hospitals, for example, work in an organizational form dedicated to advancing the state of the medical arts, in which the central currency is peer recognition and professional prestige. To be successful in such an environment, these physicians feel they need to collaborate with prestigious colleagues and believe they require new programs that will incur additional capital expenditures and increased operating costs. Presumably because such a massive effort is difficult to mount piecemeal, the tradition of the academic dowry has evolved.

Although the professional characteristics of community physicians differ somewhat from those of their colleagues in teaching hospitals, the outcome is roughly the same. Physicians in community hospitals — particularly specialists and younger physicians — have themselves been trained in the large teaching hospitals and have absorbed those institutions' emphasis upon state of the art medicine (Greer 1983). That these physicians are motivated more by practice development than research-related prestige has little effect on the outcome for the community hospital. Their desire to practice state of the art medicine inevitably engenders new programs, new capital equipment, and increased operating expenses.

From the perspective of individual patients, these decisions to develop or practice state of the art medicine are all but invisible. They are long-term decisions, which rarely if ever are affected by an individual patient's specific treatment needs. Thus, even if cost sharing could force patients to be more cost conscious and if a patient in turn could successfully transfer this cost consciousness to his or her attending physician, the resulting reduction in resource consumption (length of stay, ancillary procedures, etc.) would affect only that one patient. There is little likelihood that most physicians would carry such individual patient decisions over into their longer-run, program-based thinking. Indeed, given physicians' strong incentives to seek continuous growth at both teaching and community hospitals, the augmentation of institutional programs and facilities would most likely continue unabated despite the presence of widespread cost sharing.

In chapter 1 we disaggregated the present United States health care system into four discrete submarkets. Viewed from this perspective, cost sharing strategies seek to exert managerial control over hospitals by concentrating on only one of those submarkets, that of patients and insurers. Given the dominant role played by physicians and, to a lesser degree, by administrators in the hospital's resource allocation process, however, cost sharing's emphasis on patients is not simply incomplete, but is fundamentally misdirected. Our own field studies as well as prior research suggest that the physician/insurer and hospital/insurer submarkets hold much greater promise for effective cost containment. That is, if a cost containment strategy is to respond adequately to hospitals' existing decision-making processes, it should be aimed at those who actually make the central resource decisions.

Cost Containment and Management Control Systems

From a management perspective, this relationship between decision makers and resources is called "management control." In what is generally considered the definitive work on the topic, Anthony (1965) defines management control as "the process by which managers assure that resources are obtained and used effectively and efficiently in the accomplishment of the organization's objectives" (27). The vehicle used for carrying out management control is the management control *system,* and, although they may be called by a variety of terms, hospital reimbursement systems are de facto management control systems. That is, they are concerned with the effective and efficient use of resources by hospital managers for accomplishing a particular state's or region's objectives for hospitals.

A well-established tenet of management control theory is that a management control system has both structure and process. Structure is best thought of as the system's network of responsibility centers, that is, the individual units within an organization and their financial objectives. Managers of individual responsibility centers generally are held accountable for either revenue, expenses, profit, or return on assets, depending on the resources that the manager of each center can or should control. Thus a key task in establishing the network of responsibility centers is answering the question, Who controls which resources? In a corporate context, for example, if a manager has reasonable (not necessarily total) control over both revenue and expenses, the management control system normally will designate that manager's scope of activity as a "profit center." If only revenue is under the manager's control, then the activity is a "revenue center." And so on.

The control *process* normally consists of four interrelated sets of activities: programming, budgeting, measuring, and reporting. In a nonprofit context, the activity of evaluation frequently is included as well. Programming and evaluation generally have a multiple-year focus: programming looks ahead several years and determines the general activities the organization will engage in; evaluation looks back several years to assess how well the organization's programs have met their objectives. Budgeting and reporting, by contrast, usually focus on a single fiscal year, looking forward and backward respectively. Measurement, of course, must concern itself with the data needs for all activities. These relationships are shown schematically in figure 5.[1]

The advantage of management control theory for health care cost containment lies in its analytic focus. Although the theory was developed for industrial settings, much of it is directly applicable to current national- and state-mandated hospital reimbursement systems. To be more specific, there is in our view little conceptual difference between the management control problems posed by hospitals and those posed by large corporations with many divisions.[2] Whether by conscious design, random efforts, or studied neglect, both types of organizations always have *some form* of

Figure 5 The Management Control Process

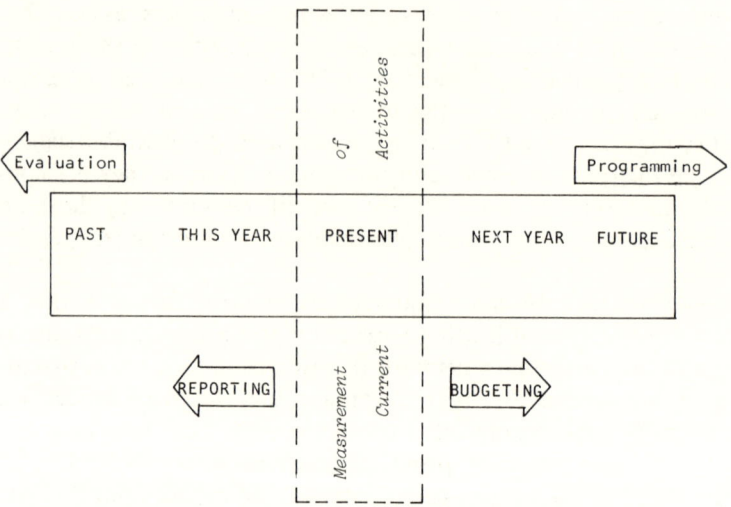

management control system in place. In some states it is a loosely structured system in which each hospital has complete autonomy; in others it exercises relatively tight control over hospitals' behavior. Nevertheless, all these approaches reflect a series of de facto management control structure and process decisions. The character of these decisions can be determined by the answers to the following questions:

Structure

- For what is a given hospital held financially responsible? Is it responsible, for example, for a fixed budget, a standard expense per patient-day, a standard expense per admission, or some other measure? [3]
- What is the relationship between the hospital and the state? To whom, for instance, do hospital-based physicians report, and for what costs (if any) are they held responsible? To whom are individual hospitals ultimately accountable: their boards of directors or a state-level agency? For what types of resource decisions are they held accountable?

Programming

- How are decisions about new programs or capital expenditures made? Individually by each hospital? By hospitals with statewide approval? Within the constraints of a statewide plan? By some other approach?

Budgeting

- How autonomous is the annual budget formulation process for an individual hospital? Does each hospital prepare its budget with minimal statewide review, or is there extensive involvement by state agencies? What resources are included in the budget, and how do they relate to the responsibility structure?

Measurement

- What type of information does each hospital collect for internal managerial purposes? What information does the state collect from individual hospitals, and how frequently?

Reporting

- What reports are regularly prepared? To whom are they distributed? What kind of action, if any, do they facilitate? What rewards or penalties exist for compliance or noncompliance with budget-determined cost ceilings?

Evaluation

- How, if at all, are individual programs in hospitals evaluated? How frequent are the evaluations? What rewards and penalties exist?

As this set of questions suggests, the hospital control systems now in place in individual states vary considerably in scope and content. Some states, particularly in the Sun Belt, have "decentralized" control systems, in which most management control takes place at the hospital (or multihospital system) level with little state oversight. Other states, mainly in the Northeast, have more "centralized" management control systems, in which hospitals must submit budgets for approval and must report regularly on a variety of compliance issues.

Centralized versus Decentralized Management Control Systems

This choice between a centralized and a decentralized system — and of course the many possibilities between these two approaches — is a crucial one for a state's cost containment efforts. As table 5 suggests, the choice must be evaluated from the perspective of both hospital programming and hospital operating decisions.

PROGRAMMING DECISIONS

As we noted above, programming decisions are generally long term in focus, looking several years into the future, and typically include new pro-

Table 5 Centralized versus Decentralized Management Control

	Type of Decision	
Type of Control	Programming	Operating
Decentralized	All programs and capital decisions other than those with major policy implications (e.g., acquisitions, divestitures) made at individual divisional (hospital) level.	Individual divisions (hospitals) responsible to corporate headquarters (state) for acceptable surplus/deficit (or return on assets) only. No cross-subsidization among divisions. No centralized budgeting.
Centralized	Program and capital decisions made by central body (e.g., corporate headquarters or the state), based on divisional (hospital) proposals.	Individual divisions (hospitals) must have operating budgets approved by corporate headquarters (state). Some cross-subsidization may take place. Divisions' financial performance is closely monitored by corporate headquarters.

grams, new services, additions of space, and new capital-equipment purchases. Programming can be, and frequently is, sporadic and ad hoc; alternatively, it can be highly routinized and scheduled; or it can contain elements of both approaches (for instance, a formal annual process for large requests with ad hoc submissions of smaller requests). A key question in each case is how much latitude individual organizational units (divisions in a multidivisional corporation; hospitals in the case of a state) are given to design and implement new programs without the review and approval of a supervising central authority (a group vice-president, corporate headquarters, or a capital budget committee of the board in the case of a large corporation; a public health department or some similar public agency in the case of a health care system). The programming aspect of table 5 thus can be further divided into type and timing dimensions, as shown in table 6.

The taxonomy in table 6 enables us to categorize the hospital programming attributes observed in the case studies in part 2. Both hospitals had moderately centralized control, but Peninsula Community had ad hoc timing whereas Oak Memorial did its programming at regular intervals. It is important to note, however, that in all cells of the matrix in table 6 the struggle to obtain resources occurred either *within* the hospital, with programs competing against other physician-generated programs, or *between* hospitals, which competed for patients against programs developed by other hospitals' physician-entrepreneurs. In no instance was there a coordinated effort, either within one hospital or between several hospitals, to

Table 6 Programming Attributes

Type of Control	Type of Control	
	Ad Hoc	Regular
Decentralized	Continuous programming at hospital level	Annual (or other interval) program planning at hospital level
Moderately centralized	Continuous programming subject to statewide approval for programs over a certain preset limit	Annual (or other interval) program planning with statewide approval for programs over a certain preset limit
Highly centralized	Continuous programming but with statewide approval for all but the smallest expenditures	Annual (or other interval) program planning with statewide approval for all but the smallest expenditures

develop the most cost effective program to meet a systemwide designated patient need. Yet such coordination is essential if the overall health delivery system is to respond effectively to an environment with increasingly limited resources.

To state the situation bluntly, in our research sites, and indeed in many states across the country, resource-allocation decisions with major social implications are being made by individual physicians and hospital administrators with little or no public input. Most of these physicians and administrators have a limited perspective on the state's overall health needs and on the most appropriate geographic distribution of health care resources. Further, many of their programming ideas and decisions reflect the constant pressure for institutional growth engendered by the present system of hospital organization and management. Certificates of need and other public restraints notwithstanding, the result has been a proliferation of duplicate (some might say "dubious") programs and unnecessary capital-equipment expenditures.

In the absence of more regularized and centralized programming systems, these kinds of program proliferation can be expected to continue, if not intensify. To suggest that the situation can be remedied by increased patient cost sharing or "systems of organized care" (HMOs) is to ignore the realities of the present physician-dominated resource allocation system. As long as society's resource decisions are left to the fragmentary and shifting needs of individual institutions' physicians and administrators, we cannot expect them to be formulated with society's best interests in mind.

In response to this difficulty, some states have opted to severely curtail the capital resources going into the system regardless of use. Such an approach can, of course, show limited short-run savings, but at what appears to be a substantial long-term cost to the viability of the system as a whole.[4] Consequently, if the United States is to reduce its hospitals' rate of expenditure increase without threatening the system's ability to provide high-quality patient care, a more centralized process for programming decisions is essential. Indeed, it is critical to the success of a redesigned hospital management control system.

OPERATING DECISIONS

A number of complexities are introduced when we move from programming decisions to operating decisions. Although the distinction between centralized and decentralized control is rather marked in the latter area, as table 5 indicates, the choice is not simple. Many multidivisional corporations have relatively decentralized control systems, for example, recognizing that divisional managers are "closest to the action" and thus need considerable latitude in decision making. By holding these managers responsible for some aggregate measure of both efficiency and effectiveness (e.g., profits or return on assets), the system motivates them to behave in what generally is believed to be the best interests of the organization as a whole. Consequently, a decentralized control system is normally selected when various divisions have highly diverse activities, when they operate in completely different markets, and of course when a single aggregate measure of *both* efficiency and effectiveness (e.g., profit) exists.[5]

Even in these situations, however, a good case frequently can be made for a more centralized management control system. The argument can be based on one of three factors: cross-subsidization, interdependence, or uncertainty. In the first instance, centralization makes it easier for an organization to cross-subsidize among its divisions. The well-known Boston Consulting Group model of stars, cash cows, and the like (Boston Consulting Group 1971) is the basis for many organizations' cross-subsidization decision making, but it requires a highly centralized control system to make the appropriate strategic trade-offs.

A second situation in which centralization is an advantage occurs when two divisions are highly interdependent, though they do not necessarily cross-subsidize each other. For example, to the extent that the Chevrolet Division of General Motors relies on the Delco Division for its batteries, an interdependence exists that requires a fairly centralized control system. At the very least, General Motors' corporate headquarters must assure itself that the two divisions are developing budgets with a consistent figure for Chevrolets' demand for batteries.[6]

Finally, in situations where external demand for a division's product or service is highly uncertain, a centralized control system generally makes sense since it allows management to measure and assess the variables that *are* under the manager's control, rather than some "all inclusive" variable such as profit. This situation usually surfaces when a division (or even a smaller organizational unit, such as a social services or medical records department in a hospital) has little or no control over the demand for its product or service. Consequently, a more centralized control system that accounts for this uncertainty (through, say, a flexible budget) is usually selected.[7]

Given these arguments for centralized management control, the case for a highly centralized budgeting and control system for hospital operating decisions is not as clear as that for capital decisions. Nevertheless, a strong case can be made for the centralized variant on the basis of all three of the factors cited above. To do so, however, we first must understand the elements that determine a hospital's cost changes between budgeted and actual expenditures or from one year to the next.

HOSPITAL COST BEHAVIOR

Most organizations, including hospitals, have three basic kinds of costs: fixed, variable, and semifixed. Fixed costs are those that remain essentially the same regardless of the number of service units delivered; the classic example is rent. Variable costs, by contrast, change almost in direct proportion to changes in the number of service units. A good example here is medication—as patient-days increase, total medication costs increase almost in direct proportion. Semifixed costs share features of both, remaining fixed over a relatively limited number of service units, then jumping to a new level; supervisory costs are perhaps the best example.[8]

Clearly, to be "ready to serve" its patients, a hospital must incur fixed costs (Feldstein 1968). Rent, administrative salaries, certain departmental personnel costs, and so forth will be present as long as its doors remain open. As patients enter the institution, however, both variable and semifixed costs are incurred. Just how is rather complex. To begin, let us assume that a given diagnosis can be expressed by the term i. If this is the case, the total amount spent (H) during any period should be the cost for each diagnosis (C_i) multiplied by the number of patients with that diagnosis (D_i). This can be expressed mathematically as

$$H = \sum_{i=1}^{n} D_i C_i .$$

If we next assume that the cost of a given diagnosis (C_i) is the cost of all resources used for that diagnosis, where R_j is a resource, and where its variable and semifixed cost is X_j, then:

$$C_i = \sum_{j=1}^{n} R_j X_j.$$

Next, if we assume that the cost of any given resource (X_j) is the cost of all units of that resource, where U_k is a unit and Y_k is its cost, then

$$X_j = \sum_{k=1}^{n} U_k Y_k.$$

To illustrate, let us take the diagnosis of ischemic heart disease (i). Treatment of such a case will require a variety of resources (R_j): the physician's time, laboratory tests, other ancillary tests (such as EKGs), hospitalization in a coronary care unit (CCU), skilled nursing care, pharmaceuticals, and so on. Each of these resources will have a cost (X_j), which is the product of the number of units (U_k) provided (hours of the physician's time, number of lab tests of each type, number of days in the CCU, etc.) and the cost (Y_k) of each of these units (physician's hourly wage, lab test rate, daily CCU rate, etc.).[9]

Adding these costs together for all necessary resources will give us the cost of treating a case of ischemic heart disease (C_i). Multiplying this total by the number of such cases in a given time period (D_i) will give us the total cost for ischemic heart disease cases for that period. Engaging in a similar process for all diagnoses will give us the total cost of care for the period.

While this model admittedly does not provide the precision its mathematical structure implies, it nevertheless gives a useful theoretical framework for answering the question, How much was spent by whom? in a given hospital. Specifically, the model makes it possible to track and monitor each component of the hospital's overall expenditures. Individual physicians in a given hospital are responsible for R_j, the resources ordered for a group of cases with the same diagnosis.[10] Similarly, the hospital's administrators are responsible for X_j, the efficient delivery of physician-ordered services. Thus, by focusing on the key actors in a hospital and the elements of the cost equation they control, the model allows us to align controllability with responsibility, a key feature of management control theory.

CENTRALIZED OPERATING CONTROL

This discussion of the hospital cost function points to several issues concerning interdependence, uncertainty, and cross-subsidization that appear to call for more centralized control than now exists in most state regulatory systems. First, with respect to interdependence, the level of fixed or standby costs needed in a given institution will depend in large measure on the type and level of standby costs incurred in other hospitals in its service area. Thus there is a high degree of interdependence in the fixed-cost decision. Second, there is uncertainty about both variable and semifixed costs, arising out of the nature of morbidity in the hospital's service area; that is, it cannot be known with certainty what types and numbers of cases will present themselves. Finally, to the extent that one hospital must serve a particularly complex or costly patient mix, there is also an element of cross-subsidization between less expensive and more expensive patients.

It therefore appears that a strong argument can be made for establishing a centralized control system for operating as well as programming decisions in hospitals. Indeed, if one relies upon the fundamental management control principles utilized by the private corporate sector, one concludes that issues of economic as well as social and political efficiency militate in favor of some form of state-level hospital managerial control. Before considering what form this control should take, however, we must examine why existing centralized hospital reimbursement systems have not been particularly effective.

Structural Failures of Existing Reimbursement Systems

Some states, particularly those with "prospective reimbursement systems,"[11] may take issue with the previous section on the basis that they already have rather centralized hospital reimbursement systems. In turn, critics of these existing systems argue that centralization of management control per se is not the cost containment solution, since states with centralized systems have been unable to demonstrate significant cost savings. Indeed, as we discussed in chapter 1, recent analyses of state rate-setting programs agree that present programs are capable of reducing annual cost increases by only a small margin. Moreover, there has been some speculation that, within the structure of present reimbursement practices, even this level of savings may not be sustainable over the long term.

ABSENCE OF MANAGEMENT CONTROL PRINCIPLES

Implicit in the discussion above is the fact that centralization of management control does not in and of itself ensure significant progress in containing overall hospital expenditures. In effect, centralization is only a necessary condition for an adequate solution, rather than its entire substance. As we discuss below, even those states with what are considered relatively sophisticated rate-setting programs have neglected several essential management control tenets.

Numerous management control theorists (Anthony 1965; Vancil 1973; Young 1979a) have argued that an effective control system must be appropriate not only to the strategy and structure of the organization it is designed for but to the behavioral incentives that characterize its decision-making processes. In the case of the hospital, therefore, a control system must be designed in light of the institution's power equilibrium and in specific response to the incentives that influence key decision-making groups within that equilibrium.

Most existing rate-setting programs, however, have not been designed with such management control criteria in mind. There are four broad categories in which we can see this absence of basic management control principles.

The first category concerns the relation between the payment unit and the resulting financial incentives for the hospital. Many state reimbursement programs at present provide hospitals with strong financial incentives *not* to act in a cost effective manner. Even prospectively oriented systems encourage the manipulation of a hospital's patient census. Specifically, in many prospective reimbursement systems, the basic unit of payment is either the traditional per diem charge or the newer per admission amount. Because these are average rates, generally including all routine care costs whether those costs are incurred in a fixed, semifixed, or variable manner, administrators have a substantial incentive to maintain patient volume at or above budgeted levels to recover fixed costs.[12]

Second, despite the shift by Medicare to diagnosis-related group (DRG) reimbursement, many prospective reimbursement systems continue to ignore the differences in resource use associated with different case types. Thus, even though they set hospital budgets in advance, these systems still facilitate cross-subsidization among both diagnostic case groups and hospital cost centers.[13] As such, they provide a limited incentive for hospital administrators to improve the efficiency with which specific services are delivered.

Third, as frequently practiced in the private sector and as adopted by state rate-setting programs, management control is predicated on a fundamentally Weberian understanding of organizational structure. The central organizing principle of this model is the hierarchical arrangement of authority, in which decision-making responsibility is centralized at the top of the organizational pyramid. As indicated in chapter 2 and demonstrated in the case studies, however, this formalistic decision-making model, with its unitary concept of organizational authority, is not well suited to the modern hospital with its two separate lines of responsibility: medical control exercised by physicians and financial control exercised by administrators. Hospital decision making, far from being controlled by "top management" at the summit of a formal organization chart, emerges from a complex pattern of compromise and conflict resolution that reflects the hospital's power equilibrium.

Inasmuch as the hospital is characterized by a conflictive rather than a hierarchical model of decision making, operating efficiency is unlikely to be significantly improved by internal management techniques that presume the existence of a single line of authority. Consequently, traditional management control tenets must be substantially revised to accommodate the hospital's nonhierarchical organization. For example, Anthony's (1965) framework is one in which "management control is a process carried on within guidelines established by strategic planning," with line managers serving as "the focal points." Likewise, Vancil (1973) is concerned about "fairness" in aligning responsibility and ability to control, and the need for what he calls "goal congruence" among the organization's responsibility centers.[14] It seems quite apparent, however, that both Anthony's guidelines and Vancil's concerns must be reconsidered for an organization in which control over resource usage is highly complex, values conflict, the definition of a "line manager" is unclear, and there is no single set of fixed organizational standards to work from.

Fourth, even the most sophisticated reimbursement programs fail to distinguish among the major cost-influencing variables in a hospital. As we indicated in the discussion of hospital cost behavior, there are essentially five variables that can explain a discrepancy between a hospital's budgeted and actual costs, or a change in its costs from one period to the next: case mix, case volume (number of cases), resources per case (mode of treatment), resource unit price, and resource delivery efficiency. Although a full discussion of this framework is presented in chapter 10, the key management control point to note here is that, far from separating managerial accountability for each of these five cost-influencing variables according to its controlling force, current state reimbursement programs typically lump all five into a single aggregate figure, for which they then hold the hospital's administration responsible. As a consequence, most existing programs make administrators accountable for costs over which they exercise minimal or no control as well as for those over which they exercise substantial control. In view of this management control lapse alone, it is not surprising that existing cost containment programs have been only marginally effective.

Implicit in this critique of existing state management control systems lies the seed of a more effective approach to hospital cost control. The five-way breakdown of hospital costs into a set of functionally and occupationally grouped variables makes it possible to discuss hospital cost inflation with considerable precision and clearly explains how present per diem reimbursement programs give hospital administrators responsibility for cost components over which they exercise only minimal control, such as case mix and resources per case. Case mix generally accounts for a significant portion of the variation in a hospital's costs, but hospital administrators exercise very little short-term control in this area. Similarly, administrators have little or no direct control over the financial consequences of physicians' patient treatment decisions. These two variables account for a substantial segment of a hospital's total expenditures, yet they are beyond the direct short-term authority of the hospital's administrators. Medicare's DRG reimbursement system has removed the effect of case mix from the administrator's responsibility but it has not directly addressed physician treatment decisions. Consequently, by making administrators responsible for physicians' decisions, DRG-based and other existing reimbursement systems persist in aggravating the fundamental tension between physicians and administrators within the hospital's power equilibrium.

At the same time, the reliance of many present reimbursement systems on per diem or per admission payments discourages administrators from efficiently managing those cost-influencing variables that *are* under their direct control, namely, resource unit price and resource delivery efficiency. By lumping these and other cost-influencing variables into one aggregate rate, existing systems obscure the effect that managerial efforts *can* have on overall cost patterns. Further, a single fixed rate encourages the administrator to concentrate less on resource price and efficiency and more on increasing the hospital's patient census to cover total operating costs. As a result, administrators may elect to concentrate on admitting patients and filling beds rather than on making their institutions more financially efficient, since the former will produce a greater total return for an equivalent effort. Thus, although this relationship may help explain administrators' emphasis on patient-generating activities (such as direct marketing, community outreach programs, and occupational health programs), it also supports the contention that present reimbursement systems do not encourage them to concentrate on the important question of organizational efficiency.

ABSENCE OF FAIRNESS AND GOAL CONGRUENCE

As we suggested above, one likely explanation for the inappropriate structure of present reimbursement systems can be found in the hierarchical character of traditional management theory in general and Vancil's (1973) two fundamental management control criteria (fairness and goal congruence) in particular. To the extent that state regulatory agencies accommodate neither the anomalous nature of the hospital's decision-making structure nor the limited authority hospital administrators have over costs, they have directly violated Vancil's two principles. By holding the administrator responsible for the financial consequences of the hospital's case mix, for example, or the costs associated with the mode of patient treatment, reimbursement systems obscure the relation between control and responsibility, thereby violating Vancil's fairness criterion. Furthermore, when they induce the administrator to meet fixed costs by encouraging physicians to extend the average length of patient stay, to increase elective admissions with high revenue/cost ratios, or to hospitalize patients who could be treated less expensively as outpatients, reimbursement systems foster unnecessary inpatient care. In such instances the goals of the individual hospital manager may well run contrary both to physicians' clinical goals and to regulators' goals for the health care system as a whole, thereby violating Vancil's goal-congruence criterion.

Summary

Present reimbursement systems encourage hospital administrators to increase patient census to cover fixed costs (or to increase the flow of discretionary revenue once fixed costs have been covered) and hold administrators accountable for many hospital costs over which they cannot exercise effective control. As a result, the three variables that can be managed at the hospital level — resources per case, resource efficiency, and (to some extent) unit prices — are not being adequately controlled, while at the same time the hospital is penalized for adverse changes in its case mix, over which it has far less control.[15] These observations about the limitations of existing systems lead one to conclude not only that greater centralization is needed in most states' reimbursement and control systems, but that much more attention needs to be paid to incorporating management control principles into the design of these systems.

Thus far we have presented little detail on exactly how greater system centralization might be structured or how management control principles might be more usefully applied. Although each state that develops a more centralized control system will need to consider a variety of factors unique to its own situation, some broad guidelines can be laid out. These are the subject of the final chapter.

CHAPTER 10
Realigning Regulatory Control

We have thus far made three essentially parallel arguments. First, on an "industry" level, we contend that the health sector has too complex a structure to be adequately supervised by market-based solutions such as increased patient cost sharing. Second, on a "firm" level, we have demonstrated that hospitals, far from being unified hierarchical organizations, are governed by an internal power equilibrium in which physicians are dominant. Finally, in the preceding chapter, we suggested that public regulatory systems — particularly hospital reimbursement systems — are de facto management control systems and that the failure of existing state regulatory attempts to control hospital cost increases reflects in substantial part flaws in their management control structure and process.

With this chapter, we wish to draw together these various conceptual strands. We do not believe that either increased state regulation, defined as more of the same, nor strategies based on cost sharing, defined in simplistic demand/supply terms, will work. What we *do* advocate is a reconceptualization of the whole hospital cost containment problem, reflecting the need to design public management control systems that can harness the hospital's power equilibrium. Precisely because hospital expenditures are generated in such a complex and interactive fashion, a successful response will require a sophisticated and flexible application of private sector management control theory to public sector social goals. Consequently, we believe there must be major realignments in the structure of existing regulatory efforts to accommodate both hospital programming and ongoing operating budgets. In the pages that follow, we present the basic outline of these realignments.

The Management Control Structure

As we noted in chapter 9, the central factor that determines the structure of a management control system lies in the question, Who controls which resources? Answering this question and then selecting an appropriate management control structure is rarely an intuitively obvious exercise, since it frequently is not clear who actually has effective control over specific resources. Moreover, choosing activities around which to organize the control structure may be difficult. Should a sports medicine program in a hospital outpatient department be a responsibility center, or should the outpatient department itself be the responsibility center? Perhaps both should be responsibility centers. If so, who should be held accountable for the resources involved in housekeeping, medical records, and other service activities?

To date, most hospital management control systems have paid insufficient attention to an appropriate alignment of responsibility and control. In large part this failure arises because different actors in the health care system control different resources. Although many actors and resources come together in the hospital, the specific relationships among them — the Who controls which resources? question — have not been carefully distinguished. The result is an ineffective management control structure.[1]

COST-INFLUENCING VARIABLES AND
THEIR CONTROLLING FORCES

An appropriate alignment of responsibility and control requires an assessment of the factors that influence costs in a hospital, followed by an analysis of which individuals control those factors. These relationships were discussed in chapter 9 and are shown schematically in table 7. By categorizing the cost-influencing variables in this way and assessing the controlling factors, we can identify the effect of each variable on a hospital's total costs and thus design a control system structure that ties these costs to those individuals within the hospital who can control them.

This series of relationships allows us to address a central cost containment dilemma that hospitals now face. Specifically, as we discussed in chapter 9, hospital administrators in many states are under intense external pressure to contain their costs, yet there are major cost-influencing variables over which they have little or no control. When we disaggregate a hospital's expenditures according to the five variables contained in table 7, it becomes apparent that hospital administrators themselves exercise direct control over only one of them, and some control over two others. The remaining variables are controlled either by physicians or by factors external to the hospital.

The first variable, case mix, is particularly complex, since it is influenced by a wide variety of demographic, epidemiologic, and fixed institutional factors (Lave and Lave 1971; Lave and Reinhardt 1976; Feldstein and Schuttinga 1977). With regard to fixed institutional factors, administrators increasingly seek to affect the composition of the medical staff, the development of new programs, and the availability of various services and facilities in an effort to alter the character of their institutions' case mix and to increase the number of elective admissions. Physicians, of course, exercise some short-range influence over elective admissions through their patterns of patient referral (Wennberg 1977), and they also exert substantial long-term or "lagged" influence over the scope of services available at

Table 7 Controlling Forces over Cost-Influencing Variables

Cost-Influencing Variable	Controlling Force			
	Environment	Physicians	Administrators	Third-Party Payers
Case mix	MUCH	Some	Little	Little
Number of cases	MUCH	Some	Some	Little
Inputs per case (mode of treatment)	None	MUCH	Little	Little
Input unit price	Some	None	Some	Little
Input efficiency	Little	Little	MUCH	Little

Source: Young and Saltman (1983a).

any given institution. In the short run, however, physicians' or administrators' influence on the hospital's *overall* case mix appears to be minor in comparison with environmental factors and prior programming decisions. Hence, cost changes due to variations in case mix should be the responsibility of third-party payers rather than persons inside the hospital. In fact, the idea that hospitals cannot control case mix in the short run is one of the basic underpinnings of DRG-based reimbursement systems.

For similar reasons, financial responsibility for the second cost-influencing variable — number of cases — also should be assigned to third-party payers. It is precisely these kinds of unknown eventualities that are covered by insurance in other sectors of society, and it seems entirely appropriate for case mix and volume changes to become the responsibility of insurers (third-party payers) in the health care system as well.[2]

The third variable, inputs per case or mode of treatment, refers to the mix of hospital resources used to treat different cases, including the patient's length of stay. Since factors such as the nature and number of laboratory tests, radiological procedures, and other ancillary services ordered for a particular admitting diagnosis are up to the physician, as is the treatment mode selected for a particular diagnosis (medication therapy, surgery, level of nursing care, etc.), control over this variable appears to rest almost exclusively with attending physicians. Thus, a more effective management control system should allocate cost containment responsibility in this area to physicians.

Last, both input unit prices and efficiencies are categories composed of costs generated by the actual production of ancillary and support services within the hospital and are the only cost factors that appear to be directly under the control of the hospital's administrators. Even here, however, external factors have a major impact on many of the hospital's unit prices.

In structural terms, then, it becomes apparent that cost containment responsibility in a properly designed hospital control system should be divided among three groups. Costs arising from case mix and number of cases should be assigned to external third-party payers; those stemming from hospital resources used per case should be assigned to the attending physician; and only those costs incurred in the actual production of hospital services should be the responsibility of the hospital's administrators.

THE AUTHORITY STRUCTURE

To design an appropriate structure for a hospital's control system, we must go beyond this formal alignment of cost-influencing variables and controlling agents. Such formal allocations of responsibility do not capture the multifaceted power relations subsumed under what we have called the hospital power equilibrium. If this realigned regulatory system is not to repeat the structural error of existing systems, therefore, we must ensure that its management control structure reflects the unofficial realities that govern most hospitals' resource allocation processes. As we discussed in chapter 2, a hospital's power equilibrium is central to its authority structure and thus must be considered in terms of the control system as well. Again, we can apply the management control lessons of the private sector to the unique world of the hospital power equilibrium.

Management control in the private sector, as we noted in chapters 2 and 9, is predicated on a fundamentally Weberian understanding of organizational structure. The central organizing principle of this model is the hierarchical arrangement of authority, in which decision-making responsibility is centralized at the top of the organizational pyramid. Barnard's (1938) definition of an organization as a group of individuals bound together by a common purpose with a set of agreed-upon goals, and his thesis that a good manager creates a "zone of indifference" within which employees strive to reach those goals, attest to the centrality of Weber's notion of authority for contemporary organization theory.

Barnard's work was seminal in the development of modern management theory. Such well-known texts as Lawrence and Lorsch's *Organization and Environment* (1967) and Andrews's *The Concept of Corporate Strategy* (1980) followed Barnard's lead in assuming a unitary hierarchical model of organizational decision making. Lawrence and Lorsch provide us with a particularly interesting example in that they adhere to this Weberian model even as they address issues of organizational decentralization. Although there have been numerous attempts to soften the impact of this unitary hierarchical model,[3] the Weberian conception of organizational authority still retains a firm grasp on the mainstream of contemporary management control theory.

As the case studies indicate, this highly formalistic model, with its hierarchical concept of organizational authority, is not well suited to modern hospitals, which are characterized by two separate lines of responsibility: medical and financial. As a consequence, operating efficiency is unlikely to be significantly improved by internal management techniques that presume the existence of a single line of organizational authority. Consequently, the determination of the *management control structure* must accommodate the hospital's nonhierarchical *organizational structure*.[4]

One recent development within management theory that may better suit the hospital's structure is matrix theory, an approach developed for organizations that operate with two simultaneous yet distinct lines of decision-making responsibility. In most matrix organizations, one line of responsibility encompasses functional department managers while the other contains "project managers" who shepherd a specific project through the "production process." Although matrix theory was initially developed in the aerospace industry to manage the complexities of large high-technology projects, it has since been successfully applied in a number of other private and public sector organizations.[5] Indeed, several commentators have proposed that a matrix system might be helpful in aligning clinical, teaching, and research functions within academic medical centers.[6]

Of particular interest is Neuhauser's (1972) suggestion that a matrix model be developed that could allocate financial responsibility for hospital costs related to patient care. A model like this might provide a structure within which an administrator would exercise financial authority over functional departments (e.g., radiology and nursing) and the attending physician would be accountable for the management of specific patient cases — what is comparable in the aerospace industry to the project under construction.[7] This format, of course, dovetails nicely with the management control principle of responsibility/control alignment discussed in chapter 9.

From a somewhat more theoretical perspective, the organizational conditions that matrix theory was designed to satisfy are clearly evident in hospitals. Specifically, according to Davis and Lawrence (1977), an organization must face three central difficulties before considering a matrix approach.[8] First, there must be two or more critical sectors of operation that require a continuous flow of simultaneous decisions. Second, the organization must operate in an unpredictable environment within which many decisions require large amounts of highly specialized knowledge, thereby forcing broadly decentralized decision making. Third, there must be strong external pressure to achieve substantial economies of scale and to utilize personnel more efficiently while still maintaining a high-quality product.

In all three respects, the modern hospital fits these conditions: (1) It requires coordination between the attending physician's medical decisions and a variety of simultaneous nonmedical activities. (2) It must be prepared to deal with any medical contingency, frequently ones requiring highly specialized medical knowledge. (3) It is under great external pressure to perform more efficiently while maintaining high-quality care.

A matrix-based managerial approach thus appears compatible with the present structure of hospital decision-making authority. Ideally, such a management approach could provide a flexible framework that would incorporate the hospital's two separate lines of authority but then hold each actor responsible for the resources over which he or she exercises control. The mechanisms by which such a system might function are described in the next section.

The Management Control Process

As we explained in chapter 9, the management control process consists of two principal activities—programming and operating. The former category has a relatively long-term focus, generally involving substantial commitments of organizational resources. The latter typically has an annual focus and includes budgeting, measuring, and reporting—supplemented in certain nonprofit organizations by evaluation.

PROGRAMMING ACTIVITIES

The programming process in teaching and community hospitals alike encompasses a wide variety of activities and can have a profound effect on health care. In the short term, the programming event—be it a new program, additional space or equipment, or the renovation of existing space—results in operating costs that go well beyond the depreciation and interest expenses of the capital resources used. New personnel, additional supplies, expansion of support service activities (e.g., housekeeping), and the like all add to the overall cost. In the long term, the new activity is likely to have secondary and tertiary effects not only directly on operating costs, but on subsequent programming activities, which then give rise to a further set of new operating costs. The result is a continuing spiral of escalating health care costs.

The findings of the case studies, coupled with prior research about capital costs, suggest the need for major changes in the programming process in most states. First, as we argued in chapter 9, we believe that both programming and operating decisions should be centralized at the state level. This means that all programming, regardless of apparent initial cost, should be subjected to meaningful public sector scrutiny and approval. Second, and equally important if a state's health care system is to have an adequate distribution of services, the public sector should take the lead in initiating necessary programming improvements through a request-for-proposal procedure.

Beyond these two bedrock elements, a proper hospital management control system must judiciously confront internal pressures generated by the hospital power equilibrium with sound and effective external review. In many multidivisional corporations a useful tension exists between individual divisions and corporate staff concerning approval of program requests, and the same type of tension could exist in a state. In many corporations, divisions are required to submit program requests to corporate headquarters for substantive and strategic review, discussion, and possible approval. Vancil and Lorange (1975) have indicated that this process is most effective when corporate headquarters has first signaled its broad priorities to the divisions, to enable them to respond to those priorities in their program submissions.

If a corporation has too many divisions to permit the smooth functioning of a direct corporate/division relationship, intermediate groups are often established as filtering mechanisms. General Electric, among other corporations, is managed in this group-based fashion. Similar mechanisms could be established in states with a large number of hospitals. The groupings may be based either on internal hospital characteristics (as some states now do for reimbursement purposes), on geography, or on other criteria.

Given the importance of program initiation and review, along with the potential for "regulatory capture" encountered by past certificate of need programs, the most appropriate regulating authority would appear to be a semiautonomous public agency, with a substantial degree of independence from the governor and the legislature. In this regard, agencies like the Food and Drug Administration or the Federal Reserve Board might be considered as prototypes.

Among their other tasks, these new semiautonomous public agencies must develop criteria to distinguish between *developing* and *practicing* state of the art medicine. Although these activities may be formally funded by different sources (federal or private grants for development and state-controlled reimbursement for practice), they are highly interrelated, as the case studies show. States need not become involved in activities directly related to medical research, although more stringent state regulation appears necessary to ensure that new technologies are diffused in a manner and at a rate consistent with the state's health care policy. Previous research has indicated that there are two very different types of problems in the deployment of new medical technology. First, it may become widely employed before its effectiveness has been fully determined and may subsequently be discontinued (Greer 1983; Fineberg 1979). Second, new medical technology, for many of the reasons described in parts 1 and 2, may be adopted in far more institutions than is justified by total patient demand (Relman 1980a; Greer 1983). Both of these technology diffusion issues can be addressed directly through an integrated and coordinated statewide programming process with a mandate to evaluate, among other things, the implementation of new medical technology.

We further believe that an adequately staffed, coordinated, and proactive programming process may obviate many of the problems associated with dowries in teaching hospitals. To ensure success, however, it is essential that the scope of monitored activities include additions to plant, structural renovations, acquisition of both new *and* replacement equipment, and new program development. There obviously is a fine line between programming activities that have purely a research function and those that have near-term implications for the cost of delivering patient care. Not only will states need to be judicious in making this distinction, but they will need to ensure that hospitals develop sufficiently sophisticated cost accounting systems to deal with the problem of allocating joint costs among teaching, research, and clinical care.[9]

We do not doubt that new public programming systems will face some initial difficulties in striking a satisfactory balance between the broad concerns of a state agency and the strategic and technical knowledge concerning patient need possessed by physicians and hospital administrators. Seeking such a balance is not unique to health care, however. Similar problems typically exist in any large organization, and they always present a difficult managerial task from both programming and operating perspectives. Much as physicians have professional, financial, and personal reasons to develop new programs, so too do most divisional and departmental managers in multidivisional corporations. The increased internal power derived from physicians' control over medical uncertainty represents a distinction of degree rather than kind. Thus, one of the very real challenges for any effective programming process is to formulate and implement its decision criteria in a way that benefits the organization as a whole.[10] That it is perhaps more difficult to establish such a process for hospitals than for other types of organizations does not make such a resolution impossible, but it does mean that greater skill is required to design a successful framework.

As the discussion above suggests, developing a coordinated public programming system, capable of achieving a satisfactory balance between public and institutional needs, will not be easy. The difficulties encountered by previous health area regulatory programs, and indeed the potential for regulatory capture in all public sector efforts to guide private sector activities, must temper any health planner's enthusiasm for such endeavors. We believe, however, that states have little real choice. As is vividly demonstrated by the case studies, *not* to engage in a serious and sophisticated regulatory effort is to simply abandon health care cost containment efforts at their most basic level. To ignore the fundamental forces that drive hospital costs, and to convince oneself that instituting "caps" on capital or turning the entire decision-making process over to so-called market forces will suffice, is to assure the continued allocation of scarce health resources according to a hospital's financial acumen, marketing prowess, and physician-dominated power equilibrium rather than the needs of the population. There is, in short, no socially acceptable alternative to a more effective state-based hospital programming process.

OPERATING ACTIVITIES

On the operating side, an effective hospital control system must be constructed from three crucial building blocks: a realistically disaggregated analysis of how hospital costs are incurred, an accurate assessment of the controlling force or forces behind each cost factor, and a sophisticated understanding of the incentives that influence key occupational groups' decision preferences within the hospital's power equilibrium.

We described the various occupational group incentives that affect the hospital's power equilibrium in chapter 3 and then gave these incentives empirical substance in the case studies. In preceding sections of this chapter, we disaggregated the hospital's total expenditures into five functionally related groupings to indicate the relation between each cost-influencing variable and its controlling agent. What remains to be done, therefore, is to outline the elements of an operating system that will associate the particular behavioral incentives of key occupational groups with the movement of particular hospital cost components.

The structure of this new control system is based on the distribution of managerial authority delineated in table 7. As we argued earlier, given this existing distribution of managerial "zones of control," an effective hospital control system should hold administrators directly responsible only for those two variables that they control: resource unit price and resource efficiency. Responsibility for the other three factors should be allocated to the appropriate controlling agents, with mode of treatment the responsibility of the attending physician and case mix and case volume the exclusive responsibility (under the present system of medical insurance) of third-party payers.

Of the several distinctions between this proposed control (or reimbursement) system and present systems, the most striking (and the most potentially controversial) is the incorporation of the attending physician into the hospital's formal management structure. Although this change is crucial to the construction of a more effective hospital control system for operating activities, it must be framed very carefully if it is not to seriously impair physicians' medical autonomy. In particular, any new effort to make physicians responsible for the financial consequences of their medical decisions raises the danger that a badly designed system might limit their ability to provide patients with the best available care. If physicians are not to be placed in an ethically untenable position, therefore, a new hospital reimbursement system must continue to provide them with maximum medical flexibility while ensuring sufficient pressure to encourage them to temper their medical judgments with a concern for the financial implications.

A primary advantage of the matrix-based control system described in the structure section is that it is fully capable of integrating this requirement for medical autonomy with the regulator's parallel requirement for overall hospital financial accountability. Precisely because decision-making responsibility is bifurcated into medical and financial lines of authority, the hospital already functions as a de facto matrix.

There are two major distinctions, however, between the hospital's existing matrix and that necessary for an effective control system. First, in the present format, one of the hospital's two lines of authority, the medical, functions almost entirely outside the financial management structure of the institution. Second, in the present framework there is no higher organizational authority — no "top management" — that exercises strategic and operational control over both administrators and physicians. Although this top management role is formally vested in the hospital's board of trustees, most boards rarely engage in the close operating control typically exercised by the chief operating officer of a private sector corporation.[11]

Thus, the two most critical changes necessary to convert a matrix-based *structure* into a matrix-based *control system* are the ability to integrate the physician into the hospital's formal management structure and the establishment of an effective hospital top management in a manner consistent with the continued delivery of quality medical care.[12]

Integrating Physicians into Hospital Management

Integrating physicians into a hospital's formal management structure can be accomplished by involving them in both budgeting and reporting. As part of the annual budgeting process, each hospital's medical staff, as a group, would be responsible both for establishing a schedule of cost-related treatment standards (what might be called "clinical treatment protocols") for each significant diagnosis in their institution and for actively monitoring their peers to ensure sufficient compliance. In this regard it should be noted that, under our proposed system, these treatment standards would be based on a national or statewide prototype but could vary from institution to institution based on a peer review process at the statewide regulatory level. Like all standards, the procedures prescribed would not necessarily be rigidly adhered to in all circumstances. Instead, the standards would serve as a guide for each physician's patient-management decisions, and their implementation could be supplemented by analysis of financial variances over a large number of cases both to identify physicians who are consistently above or below the norm and to assess the reasons why.

Such an overtly managerial and financial focus clearly involves a major shift in emphasis for most physicians. By demanding continuous management responsibility, this new management control system represents a quantum leap beyond the present short-term participation of physicians in the development of broad patient-management categories such as those incorporated into utilization review procedures or the "model treatment" screens of some private insurers (Kaplan 1980). Particularly for attending physicians, then, this new hospital control system would require a substantial change in their hospital role.

Precisely because of its mixture of financial and medical concerns, our management control proposal can be expected to evoke strong initial resistance from some physicians. Fearing that managerial responsibility ultimately would place them in the position of directly rationing access to care or of compromising their treatment modes, physicians may feel that this system could force them to weaken their professional and ethical obligation to their patients. Thus, some physicians may resist this new role not only because it involves a major new burden, but also because they see it as a threat to their professional integrity.

The success of the entire management control system, however, depends heavily on the willingness of attending physicians to accept this new managerial role. Therefore the two key questions for the success of this proposed system become: What is the incentive for attending physicians to participate in this effort? Why should they temper their medical responsibility to patients with financial responsibility to the hospital?

The answer lies in the present financial dilemma of the hospital. Essentially, physicians have little alternative to such involvement if they expect to retain full medical control over patient management. Given hospitals' current financial and political situation, a convincing argument can be made that the principal issue for physicians has become not *whether* their hospital practice will be regulated in the interests of cost containment, but only *how* and by *whom* this will be undertaken. Ample evidence of this proposition can be seen in the growing interest in DRG reimbursement systems, an interest that can only be accelerated by Medicare's adoption of the DRG method in late 1983. In DRG systems, financial standards per case type have been determined and have in effect established de facto medical treatment standards for physicians' hospital practices. Furthermore, some newer providers — such as health maintenance organizations — have rigorous programs requiring physicians to meet externally imposed performance standards that emphasize the quantity rather than the quality of care provided.[13]

Experiments have shown that physicians are both willing and able to take a more active role in the financial aspects of patient management (Hoey et al. 1982; Eisenberg 1982), although great importance generally is attached to financial incentives (Relman 1980a; Eisenberg and Williams 1981; Stone 1980a) or sanctions (Eisenberg and Rosoff 1978). Nevertheless, perhaps the most persuasive argument for physicians full cooperation with a matrix-based hospital control system is that it is the least medically intrusive of the options available. Compared with other cost containment systems such as DRGs, this new system gives physicians the opportunity to establish their own institutional standards for treatment modes, to monitor their own performance in light of those standards, and, most important, to modify their cost-inducing behavior in the manner they deem most appropriate. In effect, this management control framework lets each physician strike an essentially personal balance between the benefits of the best available treatment and the costs of providing that treatment. Moreover, this system does so without in any way holding physicians responsible for cost-influencing variables beyond their direct control — specifically, case mix, volume, efficiency, or price. By preserving their professional autonomy and by providing them with the opportunity to ensure that the mandated patient treatment standards are medically as well as financially appropriate, this alternative control system works directly to the long-term benefit of all attending physicians.

Establishing Effective Hospital Top Management

The capacity of a properly designed hospital management control system to contain costs satisfactorily without restricting patients' access to quality care hinges upon its ability to redirect the hospital's power equilibrium in a more socially suitable direction. As we postulated in chapter 2, this change requires the introjection of publicly defined goals into the ongoing workings of each hospital's decision making, such that both physicians and administrators will find voluntary compliance with new, limited-growth public mandates to be in their *own* occupational group interest.

We believe that assigning the managerial responsibility for the third cost-influencing variable, input per case, to a hospital's physicians takes a major step in co-opting the hospital's power equilibrium. Once physicians' accountability for medical practice decisions has been separated and rationalized, effective top management for the hospital can be established through a hierarchical relationship somewhat more similar to that found in other organizations. In particular, top management, working in conjunction with individual department managers, can now take responsibility for the two cost-influencing variables that are reasonably under its control: efficiency and unit prices. If, however, this new system is to be effective, it must have the following features: a redesigned cost accounting structure, a realigned management responsibility system, a variance-based reporting system, and a process of peer monitoring among physicians.

REDESIGNED COST ACCOUNTING STRUCTURE

Of central importance to this matrix-based control system is an accounting structure that clearly distinguishes among fixed, semifixed, and variable costs. Because fixed costs are related to time rather than to volume, they should be negotiated annually as a flat amount and reimbursed monthly at one-twelfth the negotiated total *regardless of patient volume*. Not only does this process force regulators to confront directly the desired level of readiness-to-serve capacity, it also removes a major incentive that administrators currently have to maintain patient-days (or admissions) at or above budgeted levels to fully recover fixed costs.

Semifixed costs associated with routine care should be negotiated in step-function fashion, with each step determined by the additional readiness-to-serve costs associated with fairly sizable increments in volume.[14] Variable costs associated with routine care should be the only costs negotiated on a per diem basis. These costs (e.g., routine care supplies and meals) can be expected to change in direct proportion to patient volume and should be reimbursed accordingly. In effect, then, for both semifixed and variable costs the hospital would be at risk for changes in unit prices, wage rates, and efficiency (changes that are controllable by the administrator) but would not be at risk for those changes that are related to case mix, volume, or physician orders.

Reimbursement for semifixed and variable costs of clinical care should be similar to that for routine care. The principal difference is that in addition to negotiating volume-based changes, the hospital and its regulatory body also would negotiate clinically based (i.e., case mix) changes. Here each hospital would use its physician-determined clinical treatment protocols for each of the institution's major diagnoses, including a physician's fee component.[15] Thus, for clinical care costs the hospital's reimbursement would depend on both volume and case mix. As with routine care costs, the hospital would not be at risk for cost changes associated with changes in case mix or volume, but its physicians would be held accountable for explaining treatment patterns that consistently exceeded or fell below the established protocols for each diagnosis. As with routine care, the hospital's administrators would be held accountable for delivering the clinical services at agreed-upon levels of efficiency and unit prices, with the hospital at risk for costs that diverged from these standards.

REALIGNED MANAGEMENT RESPONSIBILITY SYSTEM

By aligning the hospital's routine and clinical care costs with the individuals who exercise control over them, we can more effectively hold those individuals responsible for their cost-inducing behavior. In what is a considerably more comprehensive approach to the design of hospital control systems than now exists, we can assign responsibility for input unit prices and efficiency to administrators, inputs per case to attending physicians, and case mix and case volume to third-party insurers,[16] while utilizing the mandatory character of state reimbursement systems to supervise the performance of each group within its area of designated responsibility. Moreover, with an understanding of the incentives that motivate each key managerial group, state regulators can design a range of disciplinary sanctions that will directly address each group's fundamental interests.

VARIANCE-BASED REPORTING SYSTEM

A regular and timely reporting process is an essential ingredient in this matrix-based management control system. Reports must be prepared that compare actual performance with the standard, analyze the reasons for the variance between the two, and relate each variance to the responsible individual or entity. Such a reporting process would need to identify the elements shown in table 8. Within this process, for instance, physicians' performance as project managers could be routinely evaluated through both utilization review and variance analysis, and appropriate steps could be taken should they consistently use resources either above or below the clinical treatment protocols for particular case types.[17]

PEER MONITORING AMONG PHYSICIANS

At the clinical level, physicians' ordering patterns would be compared by diagnosis with the clinical treatment protocols. Physicians whose clinical ordering patterns consistently exceeded the hospital's protocol for that diagnosis would be required to provide medical justification for the observed variance. If such justification was inadequate, the physician

Table 8 Structure of Variance Analysis

Cost Element	Variance	Responsibility
Routine care, fixed cost	Actual versus one-twelfth of negotiated level	Hospital
Routine care, semifixed cost	Actual versus level determined by step	Insurers for volume changes; hospital for price and efficiency changes
Routine care variable cost	Actual versus standard (predetermined rate multiplied by volume)	Insurers for volume changes; hospital for price and efficiency changes
Clinical care, semifixed and variable costs	Actual versus level determined by combination of diagnosis, standardized clinical protocol, efficiency, and price	Insurers for case mix and volume changes; physicians for treatment protocol changes; administrators for price and efficiency changes

Source: Young and Saltman (1983b).

would be subjected to a series of professional sanctions, beginning with a written reprimand from his or her service chief and culminating, in extreme cases, in a mandatory termination of all third-party reimbursement. Because professional incentives play such a prominent role in the behavior of most physicians — and because professional concerns ultimately are so closely allied to financial concerns for salaried and fee for service physicians alike — professionally focused sanctions are quite likely to have the necessary management control impact.

Advantages of a Matrix-Based Control System

The effectiveness of a matrix approach to a hospital's organizational structure can be substantially improved by combining its basic theoretical thrust with a responsibility-focused breakdown of hospital costs. Of particular importance is the fact that controls can be instituted with minimal direct interference in the clinical decisions of the attending physician and thus with minimal adverse consequences for the overall quality of medical care the hospital can deliver.

By adding this structural and behavioral dimension to the functional analysis described in table 7, we can develop a management control system that can pinpoint the probable cause as well as the likely source of a particular expenditure. Moreover, by separating fixed from nonfixed costs, the reimbursement system can guarantee a hospital a negotiated level of fixed obligations annually, thereby removing a major incentive for the hospital administrator to increase the institution's patient census.

Such a control and reimbursement system, by addressing the management problem created by the hospital's power equilibrium, offers substantial cost containment advantages both to the hospital and to state regulatory authorities. By recognizing and incorporating the hospital's nonhierarchical pattern of authority, the new system can better accommodate the highly segmented way a hospital actually incurs costs. Areas of managerial responsibility that rest with administrators and physicians inside the hospital can be distinguished from those that belong to third-party payers. Moreover, all cost responsibility can be properly assigned, monitored, and managed. By restricting administrators' zones of responsibility to those areas they can control, this revamped system makes administrative efforts more visible and thus encourages more cost effective behavior.

Furthermore, by bringing attending physicians into the control system and thereby inducting them into the formal managerial structure of the hospital, this new control system responds to the existence and character of the hospital power equilibrium. This change is important for the hospital's long-term stability, since by ushering this key decision-making group into a position of formal authority the hospital obligates physicians to consider the needs of the institution as a whole. Properly structured and implemented, the system also can affect physicians' careers in that it generates a managerial record on each individual's overall performance, which presumably would be of interest to other hospitals to which he or she might apply for privileges. In effect, this revamped control system initiates a process of formal co-optation (Selznick 1949) that encourages physicians to temper their self-interest with a concern for the hospital.

This control system also can help counterbalance the desires of both administrators and physicians for continuous institutional growth. By disaggregating managerial responsibility along both functional and patient-management lines, and by reinforcing this breakdown through cost distinctions and variance analysis, the system generates a record of which cost-influencing variables have diverged from budget and by how much. This process of isolating individual responsibility holds promise of generating peer concern about the financial consequences for the institution as a whole. It also permits state regulatory authorities to assess more clearly the reasons for increases in hospital operating costs and to begin to perform some of the top management tasks that are all but neglected under present reimbursement systems.

Conclusions

Matrix-based management control supplemented by effective program review and approval within a centralized system gives both regulators and hospital administrators the tools necessary to fashion effective cost containment programs. The ability to integrate the hospital's growth and development strategy with the structure of its reimbursement and control process lets regulators minimize the number of perverse incentives within the system. Additionally, by placing the key actors in the hospital's power equilibrium in positions of direct management responsibility, a matrix system can help reduce the structural conflict between the interests of the hospital's occupational groups and its cost containment efforts.

We must recognize, however, that even the most accurately targeted management control system cannot by itself accomplish the entire cost containment task. The endeavor will require substantial support from the broader medical, cultural, and political realms of society that reinforce particular notions of professional and institutional success. In this regard we wish to return to the issue of cost sharing versus regulation.

With this book we have sought to present the case for a more effective regulatory strategy for hospitals. We believe that a centralized state control system, using a matrix approach to hospital cost containment, illustrates the sophisticated levels of regulatory intervention that are possible, thereby demonstrating the validity of our introductory point that it is not regulation per se that is the source of the financial crisis in the health care system, but *ineffective* regulation. Indeed, we suggest that a blind reversion to market forces not only would fail to restrain the wide range of cost-inducing factors that are beyond the control of the individual hospital, but also would not adequately address the driving forces behind the hospital power equilibrium. In particular, cost sharing and the competition it produces can be expected to continue to inhibit the evolution of an effective top management for hospitals, reinforcing the mismatch between a hospital's reimbursement structure, on the one hand, and its organizational strategy, structure, control system, and behavioral incentives on the other. Additionally, the competition for patients will further exaggerate both the dominant position of the "patient providing" physician within the hospital power equilibrium and the pernicious financial effects of existing reimbursement systems. In sum, the challenge to health policymakers is not to seek dubious mechanisms by which to justify dismantling existing regulatory apparatus, but instead to create appropriate devices to overhaul that apparatus so that it might fulfill both its intended function and its promise.

Notes

Chapter 1. The Cost Containment Challenge

1. Joskow (1981) has disaggregated the overall rate of increase into its component parts. His analysis of the reasons for cost increases between 1970 and 1979 indicates that inflation (i.e., increases in unit prices) accounted for 60 percent of the rise. The remaining 40 percent was divided between intensity of care (30 percent) and volume (10 percent). Intensity of care is defined as the "quality, quantity, and the scope of services provided."

2. One need only contrast Sweden's 1982 infant mortality rate of 6.8 percent to that of the United States — 11.3 percent overall and 19.6 percent for blacks — to grasp the fundamental character of this difference. For an assessment of the Swedish system see the chapter by Edgar Borgenhammer in Raffel (1984).

3. See Conrad and Marmor (1980) for a definition of different types of cost sharing and the arguments for and against it. See Ginzberg (1983b) for a longer discussion of market-based proposals and the analytical distinctions among them. For a different perspective, incorporating the private (corporate) sector, see Schlenker and Shanks (1983). For a good overall summary of the various proposals see Sigelman (1983).

4. Chicago *Tribune,* "Hospitals Face Closings: Costs Imperil 25 in Chicago Area, Study Says," 22 July 1984, 1.

5. On this point see Hellinger (1982).

6. For an overview of these approaches, see Joskow (1981). For a discussion of the concept of incentive-based reimbursement see Bauer and Densen (1974). For an analysis of the relation between cost and case mix see Feldstein (1965), Lave, Lave, and Silverman (1972), and Thompson, Fetter, and Mross (1975). For a discussion of prospective reimbursement and efficiency see Worthington (1976).

7. For an overview of these approaches see Kleinberg (1980).

8. Sahin and Taylor (1979) suggest in a different but related vein that large corporations may find it more cost effective to acquire their own health care facilities than to pay health insurance premiums for their employees. See Kaplan (1980) for a detailed description of the administrative structure of one such self-funded program.

9. For a general discussion on this point, see Carels (1980), Joskow (1981), and Brown (1983).

10. For a discussion of the legal history of these challenges, see Weiner (1977). For a detailed discussion of one state's experience with legal challenges to its rate setting program, see Hamilton and Kamens (1979), particularly 31-36.

11. See Brown (1983), especially 509, for a complementary perspective on this point.

12. Some of these issues are taken up in greater detail in chapter 2. See also Stern and Epstein (1985).

13. It should be noted that in other countries such direct financial pressures on hospitals appear to have been more successful in reducing hospital expenditure. Detsky et al. (1983), for example, documents the apparent success in Canada's On-

tario Province of just such a "capped" revenue structure and concludes that this form of hospital regulation can in fact work well. Beyond cultural and social issues, however, the Canadian experience reflects a number of contextual anomalies that differ from accepted policy practice in the United States. Not only did each Ontario hospital have a province-defined "global budget," but the provincial ministry of health had the legal right to step in and administer the hospital if, in Detsky's words, "management appears to be ineffective" (158). Moreover, Detsky says he cannot describe the consequences of Ontario's regulatory experience for questions of physicians' behavior, patients' health status, or interinstitutional competition — questions we believe are central to a successful cost containment effort in the United States.

Other researchers have pointed to further differences. Raffel (1984) notes that efforts on the hospital level in Canada were preceded by a successful national effort to restrain key supply factors, including the number of trained physicians, and concludes that this sequence is essential in explaining the success of global budget controls on hospitals. Additionally, the imposition of national wage and price controls during 1976 to 1979 had a dramatic effect on personnel costs. In all instances one can point to precisely the type of more centralized managerial authority in Canada that we propose in part 3 of this volume.

Chapter 2. The Hospital Power Equilibrium: A Theoretical Framework

1. For instance, see Stone (1980b), Starr (1980), and Havighurst (1980).
2. See the short case studies presented in Brady (1980) and Weiblen (1980).
3. For a general discussion see Millman (1977) and Green (1975).
4. See, for example, the case study in Keith (1980) and the discussion in Redisch (1978). Also the more general discussion in Bucher and Stelling (1969), Croog and Ver Steeg (1972), and Gordon (1964).
5. Although they are not an occupational group, there is also the hospital board of trustees.
6. The issue of motivation — of both physicians and administrators — will be taken up in greater detail in chapter 3.
7. If there is a surplus of physicians in certain specialties in a locality, or if there is increasing market penetration by alternative health delivery vehicles, like HMOs and neighborhood clinics, in which fee discipline has been imposed by placing physicians on an annual salary, a hospital's admitting physicians may find that their implicit threat to withdraw from the hospital staff no longer generates the same apprehension in hospitals administrators. We are indebted to Steven Hegarty (vice-president, health care finance, Massachusetts Hospital Association) for his observations on both this point and that in note 8.
8. In particular, boards have been willing to pursue various forms of multi-institutional collaboration despite the expressed desires of their hospitals' physicians and administrators. Also, some boards have intentionally given their senior administrators long-term employment contracts to encourage them to undertake politically difficult and organizationally painful cutbacks in services or facilities. In both these instances the net result of the board decisions has been to challenge the physicians' traditional dominance over hospital decision making.

Chapter 3. Behavioral Incentives in the Hospital Power Equilibrium

1. "Baptist Medical Center Files a Bankruptcy Petition," *New York Times,* 4 March 1981.
2. *Boston Globe,* 20 May 1981.
3. There are, of course, a few elite institutions that remain small by choice. Even these institutions, however, regularly seek to renew the quality of their facilities, equipment, programs, and medical staff and thus continue to grow on at least some of the continua noted. In fact, given inflationary trends in the economy, these institutions are also growing. See Young (1982).
4. Harris (1977) noted this tendency toward "bigness and betterment" particularly in large urban hospitals, but he ascribed this dynamic solely to the defensive needs of each chief of service for "service redundancy," not to a much more deeply ingrained set of behavioral pressures based both in the structure of the hospital's power equilibrium and in the broad societal definition of "professional success." Relman (1980b) also criticized the tendency, attributing it to a quest for profit rather than to something more basic and causal.
5. See Schroeder (1980) for a discussion on this point.
6. Ashkenas (1979) found in his study of a medical school department that the mix of these incentives can vary dramatically with the physician's age and cultural generation (pre-World War II; post-World War II, etc.). It should also be noted in this context that Ashkenas (1979), Monsma (1970), Schroeder (1980), Mechanic (1980), Brown and Marks (1981), and others have all observed that there is no absolute empirical knowledge on which influences do in fact determine specific physician decisions.
7. Schroeder (1980), for example, describes this social contract incentive as "the most common and important reason" for physicians' ordering behavior (32).
8. For a broad general analysis of this issue, see Friedson (1970).
9. Since sufficient informal pressure can lead to formal sanctions, the informal mechanisms should be perceived as a less structured and perhaps predictive component of the formal structure of physician control and regulation.
10. For a discussion of this point, see Redisch (1978).
11. This argument does not necessarily contradict the findings of researchers like Freidson (1976) who argue that physicians exercise very little collective control over the *quality* of medicine practiced by their peers. The oversight function of organized medicine seems to be to ensure that a physician's practice conforms to established professional norms in its style and form rather than in its effectiveness.
12. All of these elements, but particularly the first two, are illuminated in the case studies in part 2.
13. See Curran (1983). For one explanation of the causes of this increase, see Kotelchuck (1976, 419-39).
14. With regard to the possibility that unnecessary surgery will remain undetected by a hospital's tissue committee, one should note that Monsma's argument suggests that though a removed organ may have been diseased, the condition could have been treated medically instead of surgically.
15. We are indebted to Alfred Gellhorn, M.D., for pointing out this relationship.

16. This variance has been vividly demonstrated by Richard Freyer, M.D., former director of medical services at Prince Alfred Hospital in Sydney, Australia. Freyer found that younger physicians often had practice profiles that were substantially more costly to the hospital than those of more experienced physicians and that appropriate intervention could help make their practice styles substantially more cost effective. Freyer's work is unpublished.

17. Numerous other analysts have also commented upon the relation between institutional growth and the administrator's professional advancement. McClure (1976) linked institutional growth to the administrator's "status and prestige," and Lee (1971) argued that the hospital's status was the linchpin upon which all of the administrator's rewards—salary, security, reputation, personal satisfaction—were based. Schultz and Rose (1973) similarly noted that "growth indicates the success" of the administrator's policies (5).

18. Blishen (1969) provides a good summary of professional pressures that affect nurses.

19. For a perspective analysis of the difficulties nurses have encountered in their attempts to fulfill their desires through unionization, see Levi (1980) and the discussion of unionization efforts in Krause (1977).

20. These decisions, particularly input price and input efficiency, are the responsibility of the hospital administrator. See Young and Saltman (1982) for a more detailed discussion on this point.

21. See Silvers (1981) for an interesting discussion of this linkage.

22. See Salkever and Bice (1978) for an analysis of this problem. However, even such "success" can itself become the back door through which the hospital can justify an expansion of beds. As Brown (1981) suggests, once several new quality-enhancing facilities are in place (cardiac catheterization laboratories, coronary care units, and so on), these new facilities may be able to operate at capacity only if the hospital is allowed to add to the number of available beds.

23. See La Violette (1980) for a descriptive account of how one hospital went about unbundling its various operations. Seaver (1977) provides a description of a similar set of activities.

24. Goldsmith (1980) provides a good example of such a marketing strategy. Starr (1982) also comments on these and similar activities.

25. For a dramatic illustration of the length to which these delaying tactics can be taken, see the description in Hamilton and Kamens (1979) of the downstate New York reimbursement program's legal problems during 1977 and 1978, especially 31–36.

Chapter 5. The Decision-Making Structure at Oak Memorial Medical Center

1. There were no female chiefs at Oak Memorial.

2. A "dowry" was a commitment made to a chief in order to attract him to the hospital. This practice is discussed at length in chapter 7.

3. There were no female subchiefs at Oak Memorial.

Chapter 6. Programmatic Decision Making at
Peninsula Community Hospital

1. The chief and one colleague were, as previously noted, salaried to the hospital, while the remainder of the psychiatrists were private practitioners who were reimbursed on a fee for service basis.
2. Reimbursement of renal dialysis for all patients was covered by a special adjunct to the federal Medicare program.
3. Certificate of need was required for all hospital capital projects over $150,000. The hospital was required to submit an application to the state department of public health justifying the need for the expenditure. The project could take place only if the application was approved.
4. These funds were to purchase equipment in addition to those machines already available in the operating room, where endoscopic procedures were being performed. The existing machines had been purchased as part of the department of surgery's capital requests.
5. Blue Cross pays the hospital component of a patient's stay; Blue Shield pays the physician's fee.

Chapter 7. Programmatic Decision Making at
Oak Memorial Medical Center

1. Nevertheless, within the past seventeen years, no chief had left Oak Memorial to become chief at another hospital.
2. However, the expected clinical volume was not met, and it became a "loser."
3. LCME: Liaison Committee on Medical Education (concerned with medical student education); LCGME: Liaison Committee on Graduate Medical Education (concerned with house staff education).
4. These "dips" were related to unavailability of physicians, not patients.

Chapter 8. An Analysis of the Two Power Equilibria

1. For further discussion of the utility of field research of the sort we conducted, see Young (1979b), especially chapter 2 and appendix A. Also see Christenson (1975) and Bernard (1957).
2. Although financial viability is one aspect of a large medical practice, it was not the predominant one for Peninsula's physicians. In any event, the financial return from a healthy practice may be dispersed over a long period, reflecting the illness patterns of different diseases and patients. Also, size and composition (types of illnesses treated or procedures performed) of practice itself is a form of professional prestige; that is, the power-related pecking order at Peninsula was defined by an individual physician's professional reputation in the eyes of his or her colleagues, based in this instance on practice characteristics.
3. House staff generally refers to residents and interns. Although one never sensed that Oak Memorial's chiefs felt threatened by these intradepartmental relations, the tensions certainly did not represent a source of comfort to them.

4. Recall that the dowry of Oak Memorial's new chief of medicine included substantial support to develop cardiology and gastroenterology subspecialty programs, even though several nearby teaching hospitals also possessed such subspecialty services. From this chief's perspective, however, no department of medicine could be considered complete without these subspecialties, and they thus were required if Oak Memorial was to be a prestigious medical center. In fact, Oak Memorial's chief of surgery thought these subspecialty medical programs were so important that he was willing to give up space (a key resource) to obtain them.

5. Salkever and Bice (1978) and others have shown that the approval rates for certificate of need applications are very high. This suggests either that hospitals are extremely judicious about the proposals they submit or, more likely, that the state has little real desire or ability to curtail hospital-driven development. Begley, Shoeman, and Traxler (1982) have attempted to identify some of the relevant explanatory factors.

6. Furst and Markland (1980); Brown and Marks (1981).

7. Although outpatient psychiatry was a "loser" at Oak Memorial, it was a "winner" at Peninsula Community (see table 4). The difference lies in patients' insurance status and also in patient management practices. Psychiatrists at Oak Memorial saw a generally poorer population (e.g., more Medicaid patients) and allowed patients to receive services even though their insurance coverage had been exhausted. As such, the hospital often was not compensated. This was not the intention of the new program at Peninsula Community. On the contrary, only insured patients were seen at the outpatient clinic, and in fact the insurance issue was used to encourage patients to switch out of the clinic and become private patients of Peninsula Community Hospital's psychiatrists. In effect, the outpatient clinic there was both an occupational health program necessity and a feeder of profitable private psychiatric patients, a role quite different from that of the outpatient program at Oak Memorial.

8. This behavior in part reflects the fact that the physician and the hospital are reimbursed by separate systems (Blue Shield and part B of Medicare being the two principal sources of physicians' payments). In the case of internists, the reimbursement comes as a result of a visit to the bedside: the more patients in beds, the more visits, and the greater the total reimbursement. Thus, when it is not possible to get one's patient into the hospital, the concern with length of stay (generally of other physicians' patients) may arise. In this regard it should be noted that the recent change in Medicare reimbursement policy to pay hospitals based on diagnosis-related groups does not as yet include physician payments. Thus we can expect to see the power struggle between administrators and physicians further exacerbated: administrators will be stressing the importance of an early discharge, which for the physician may mean reduced income.

Chapter 9. The Need for Centralized Management Control Systems

1. Space limitations prevent us from going into depth on management control theory in general. For a discussion of its use in industry context, see Anthony, Dearden, and Bedford (1984). For its applicability to nonprofit organizations, see

Anthony and Young (1984). For a discussion of some basic management control principles and their relationship to health delivery organizations, see Young (1984).

2. This argument is made at greater length in Young and Kane (1984).

3. See Dowling (1974) for a discussion of different payment units. In management control terms, these constitute the responsibility of the responsibility center manager.

4. See Cohodes (1983) for an analysis of this.

5. See Chandler (1962) for the classic analysis of the choice between centralization and decentralization in a corporate context. The health care parallel is discussed in Young and Kane (1984).

6. There is also the significant (and relatively complex) question of the appropriate transfer price (Solomons 1965), but the subject is beyond the scope of this book. For a discussion of the applicability of transfer pricing to a health care reimbursement context, see Young (1981).

7. See Finkler (1981) for a discussion of the use of flexible budgets in a hospital.

8. For a more complete discussion of these three cost types, see Young (1984).

9. We would become even more sophisticated by breaking down some units, such as lab tests, into their material and labor components, but this extra level of detail would complicate the analysis considerably without adding significantly to its explanatory power.

10. More specifically, they can be held responsible for the difference between some predetermined *standard* R_j and their *actual* R_j. We discuss this more fully in the next section.

11. A prospective reimbursement program seeks to limit a hospital's revenues by setting its payment rates and volume estimates in advance and holding it responsible for meeting the resulting budget. See Dowling (1974).

12. This is accomplished either through medical staff appointments or through decisions relating to elective admissions and patients' length of stay. By using these techniques, some administrators have found it possible to encourage physicians to increase total patient-days in the institution. Some prospective systems have attempted to correct for these perverse incentives by using volume corridors and reimbursing volume shortfalls in accordance with some estimate of the relation between fixed and variable costs. This estimate usually is quite arbitrary, however, and still retains the essential mistake of reimbursing fixed or "period" costs on the basis of volume.

13. The DRG approach is an attempt to correct for this sort of cross-subsidization. As Doremus (1980) has suggested, as we have argued in Young and Saltman (1982), and as Stern and Epstein (1985) demonstrate, however, the DRG approach suffers from several major drawbacks.

14. Vancil's "fairness criterion" stipulates that measures used by top management to judge a line manager's decision should be appropriate; for example, a "good" decision from the manager's perspective should lead to a "good" measurement in the control system. The "goal congruence" principle stresses the importance of structuring the control system so that actions in the best interests of a particular manager or division also are in the best interests of the entire organization.

15. As noted previously, Medicare's DRG-based reimbursement system has attempted to correct for this deficiency, but it suffers from several built-in flaws of the DRG methodology (see Young and Saltman 1982). More important, it does not attempt to distinguish among the three variables that can be managed at the hospital level and their controlling forces, a point we return to in chapter 10.

Chapter 10. Realigning Regulatory Control

1. See Young and Saltman (1983a) for additional details on this point. A notable exception is Johns Hopkins Hospital in Baltimore, which appears to have developed some useful realignments of its management control structure (see Zuidema 1980; Heyssel et al. 1984); but, as we discuss in the next section, even the Johns Hopkins model does not appear to have fully distinguished among all the "cost-influencing variables" and their controlling forces.

2. As we discussed in chapter 9, the principal reason administrators are shown as having "some" control over the number of cases is the incentives inherent in existing reimbursement systems to achieve budgeted levels of admissions or days of care in order to adequately cover the institution's fixed costs. We propose a solution for this problem later in this chapter.

3. One thinks particularly of the Human Relations School, founded by Fritz Roethlisberger and Elton Mayo, and its successors.

4. For a similar argument, see Charns, Lawrence, and Weisbord (1977).

5. For a discussion of the growth of matrix theory's uses, see Davis and Lawrence (1977). A brief description of the management control aspects of a matrix organization can be found in Jay Galbraith (1973).

6. See Davis and Lawrence (1977) and Charns, Lawrence, and Weisbord (1977).

7. This distribution of hospital responsibility would, from a managerial standpoint, serve to institutionalize the physician's role as overseer within what Bauerschmidt (1970) describes as the "individualized production unit" structure of hospital organization and Harris (1979) terms the "internal control" structure.

8. Davis and Lawrence (1977) point out some of the difficulties in developing and implementing a matrix-based organization. Both they and Anthony, Dearden, and Bedford (1984) stress the importance of exceptional leadership to induce the necessary teamwork.

9. The accounting problems of joint costs are discussed in Anthony and Reece (1983).

10. This topic has been covered in detail by a variety of management theorists. Perhaps the best discussion can be found in Bower (1970); other good sources include Lawrence and Lorsch (1967), Vancil (1973), Vancil and Lorange (1975), Cyert and March (1963), Anthony and Young (1984), and Barnard (1938).

11. Indeed, one could well argue that the importance of the hospital's power equilibrium is certainly a result, if not the cause, of this managerial void.

12. Both the emphasis on the formal integration of the physicians into hospital management and the emphasis on case management responsibility distinguish this system from that now used at the Johns Hopkins Hospital (Zuidema 1980; Heyssel et al. 1984).

13. See Carnoy, Coffee, and Koo (1976).

14. For example, a 10 percent increase in volume above that associated with the negotiated fixed-cost level would likely require additional staff for nursing, housekeeping, dietary, and so forth; these workers and other semifixed costs would be paid in accordance with an additional predetermined amount of reimbursement; and so on until the hospital's full capacity was reached. For a discussion of a system that broaches these distinctions, see Wood (1982).

15. This is an important (and currently missing) element in the system. By having a separate physician fee structure, regulators simply exacerbate the problems of the power equilibrium. Specifically, when there are two parallel reimbursement systems (hospital and physician), physicians frequently find themselves facing conflicting financial incentives.

16. We may also wish to assign some unit price responsibility to third parties, depending on the extent to which certain unit prices are truly outside the control of the hospital manager. A good example is energy prices.

17. See Anthony and Welsch (1981) for a good introductory discussion of variance analysis. For additional details, see Gordon and Shillinglaw (1974). For a discussion of its applicability to DRGs, see Soliman and Hughes (1983). It is important to recognize that an essential characteristic of variance analysis is that it does not focus on only one decision or activity. Instead it looks at gaps between standard and actual costs over a large number of activities. Additionally, it is designed to be used not as a club, but rather as a tool to assist managers in asking the appropriate questions to determine why actual costs deviated from the standard.

References

Andrews, Kenneth R. 1980. *The concept of corporate strategy.* Rev. ed. Homewood, Ill.: Richard D. Irwin.
Anthony, Robert N. 1965. *Planning and control systems: A framework for analysis.* Boston: Division of Research, Harvard Business School.
Anthony, Robert N., John Dearden, and Norton M. Bedford. 1984. *Management control systems.* 5th ed. Homewood, Ill.: Richard D. Irwin.
Anthony, Robert N., and James S. Reece. 1983. *Accounting: Text and cases.* Homewood, Ill.: Richard D. Irwin.
Anthony, Robert N., and Glenn A. Welsch. 1981. *Fundamentals of management accounting.* Homewood, Ill.: Richard D. Irwin.
Anthony, Robert N., and David W. Young. 1984. *Management control in non-profit organizations.* Homewood, Ill.: Richard D. Irwin.
Ashkenas, Ron. 1979. The behavioral sciences and physicians' concerns. *Health Care Management Review* 4 (Fall): 73–80.
Badgley, Robin F., and R. D. Smith. 1979. *Users charges for health services.* Toronto: Ontario Economic Council.
Barer, M. L., et al. 1979. *Controlling health care costs by direct charges to patients: Snare or delusion?* Toronto: Ontario Economic Council.
———. 1982. *Income class and hospital use in Ontario.* Toronto: Ontario Economic Council.
Barnard, Chester I. 1938. *The functions of the executive.* Cambridge: Harvard University Press.
Bauer, Katherine G. 1977. Hospital rate-setting—this way to salvation. *Milbank Memorial Fund Quarterly* 55 (Winter): 117–58.
Bauer, Katherine G., and Paul M. Densen. 1974. Some issues in the incentive reimbursement approach to cost containment: An overview. *Medical Care Review* 31:61–100.
Bauerschmidt, Alan D. 1970. The hospital as a prototype organization. *Hospital Administration* 15 (Spring): 6–14.
Beck, R. G. 1974. The effects of copayment on the poor. *Journal of Human Resources* 9 (Winter): 129–42.
Begley, Charles E., Milton Schoeman, and Herbert Traxler. 1982. Factors that may explain interstate differences in certificate of need decisions. *Healthcare Financing Review* 3 (June): 87–94.
Bernard, Claude. 1957. *An introduction to the study of experimental medicine.* New York: Dover.
Biles, Brian, Carl J. Schramm, and J. Graham Atkinson. 1980. Hospital cost inflation under state rate setting programs. *New England Journal of Medicine* 302 (18 September): 664–66.
Blishen, Bernard R. 1969. *Doctors and doctrines: Ideology of medical care in Canada.* Toronto: University of Toronto Press.
Boston Consulting Group. 1971. Growth and financial strategies. Boston. Mimeographed.
Bower, Joseph L. 1970. *Managing the resource allocation process: A study of*

corporate planning and investment. Boston: Division of Research, Graduate School of Business Administration, Harvard University.

Brady, Jane F. 1980. A power struggle in the department of surgery. In *Case studies in health administration,* vol. 2, ed. James O. Hepner, pp. 103–10. Saint Louis: C. V. Mosby.

Brook, Robert H., et al. 1983. Does free care improve adults' health? Results from a randomized control trial. *New England Journal of Medicine* 309 (8 December): 1426–34.

Brown, Jonathan B. 1981. Cardiac catheterization and surgery programs in Massachusetts: Capacity and economy. Unpublished manuscript, Harvard School of Public Health, Boston.

Brown, Jonathan B., and Harry M. Marks. 1981. Buying the future: The relationship between the purchase of physical capital and total expenditure growth in US hospitals. In *Health capital issues,* pp. 27–46. Washington, D.C.: Department of Health and Human Services.

Brown, Lawrence D. 1983. *Politics and healthcare organization: HMOs as federal policy.* Washington, D.C.: Brookings Institution.

Buchanan, James M., and C. M. Lindsey. 1970. Financing of medical care in the United States. In *Health services financing.* London: British Medical Association.

Bucher, Rue, and Joan Stelling. 1969. Characteristics of professional organizations. *Journal of Health and Social Behavior* 10 (March): 3–15.

Butler, Richard J., David J. Hickson, and Arthur E. McCullough. 1974. Power in the organization coalition. Paper presented at World Congress of Sociology.

Caper, Philip, and David Blumenthal. 1983. What price cost control? Massachusetts new hospital payment law. *New England Journal of Medicine* 308 (3 March): 542–44.

Carels, Edward J. 1980. Health care costs: The magnitude of the problem. In *The physician and cost control,* ed. Edward J. Carels, Duncan Neuhauser, and William B. Stason, pp. 3–21. Cambridge, Mass.: Oegeschlager, Gunn, and Hain.

Carnoy, J., L. Coffee, and L. Koo. 1976. Corporate medicine: The Kaiser health plan. In *Prognosis negative: Crisis in the health care system,* ed. D. Kotelchuck, pp. 363–86. New York: Vintage Books.

Chandler, Alfred D. 1962. *Strategy and structure: Chapters in the history of the American industrial enterprise,* Cambridge: MIT Press.

Charns, Martin P., Paul R. Lawrence, and Marvin Weisbord. 1977. "Organizing multiple-function professionals in academic medical centers. *North-Holland/TIMS Studies in the Management Sciences* 5:71–88.

Christenson, Charles J. 1975. Proposal for a program of empirical research into the properties of triangles. Working paper 75-23, Harvard Business School, Boston. Mimeographed.

Clarkson, Kenneth. 1972. Some implications of property rights in hospital management. *Journal of Law and Economics* 15 (October): 363–76.

Cohodes, Donald R. 1983. Which will survive? The $150 billion capital question. *Inquiry* 20:5–11.

Congressional Budget Office. 1981. *The impact of PSROs on health-care costs: Update of CBO's 1979 evaluation.* Washington, D.C.: U.S. Government Printing Office.

Conrad, Douglas, and Theodore R. Marmor. 1980. Patient cost sharing. In *National health insurance: Conflicting goals and policy choices,* ed. Judith Feder, John Holiham, and Theodore R. Marmor. Baltimore: Urban Institute.

Coser, Rose L. 1958. Authority and decision-making in a hospital: A comparative analysis. *American Sociological Review* 23 (February): 56-63.

Croog, Sidney H., and Donna F. Ver Steeg. 1972. The hospital as a social system. In *Handbook of medical sociology,* ed. Sol Levine and Leo G. Reeder. Englewood Cliffs, N.J.: Prentice-Hall.

Crozier, Michel. 1964. *The bureaucratic phenomenon.* Chicago: University of Chicago Press.

Curran, William J. 1983. Medical malpractice claims since the crisis of 1975: Some good news and some bad. *New England Journal of Medicine* 309 (17 November): 1107-8.

Cyert, Richard M., and James G. March. 1963. *A behavioral theory of the firm.* Englewood Cliffs, N.J.: Prentice-Hall.

Dalton, Gene W., Louis B. Barnes, and Abraham Zaleznik. 1968. *The distribution of authority in formal organizations.* Boston: Division of Research, Graduate School of Business Administration, Harvard University.

Davis, Karen. 1973. Hospital costs and the Medicare program. *Social Security Bulletin* 36 (August): 1-19.

Davis, Stanley, and Paul J. Lawrence. 1977. *Matrix.* Reading, Mass.: Addison-Wesley.

Detsky, Allan S., et al. 1983. The effectiveness of a regulatory strategy in containing hospital costs: The Ontario experience, 1967-1981. *New England Journal of Medicine* 309 (21 July): 151-59.

Dirksen, Charles J. 1978. Determining how and why your costs are changing. *Hospital Financial Management* 32 (December): 14-25.

Dolan, Andrew K. 1980. Antitrust law and physician dominance of other health practitioners. *Journal of Health Politics, Policy and Law* 4:675-90.

Doremus, H. D. 1980. DRGs may be raising false expectations. *Hospitals* 54:47-51.

Dowling, William L. 1974. Prospective reimbursement of hospitals. *Inquiry* 11: 163-80.

———. 1979. Hospital rate-setting programs: How and how well, do they work? *Topics in Health Care Financing* 6 (Fall): 15-23.

Egdahl, Richard H. 1984. Should we shrink the healthcare system? *Harvard Business Review* 62 (January-February): 125-32.

Eisenberg, John M. 1982. The use of ancillary services: A role for utilization review? *Medical Care* 20:849-61.

Eisenberg, John M., and A. J. Rosoff. 1978. Physician responsibility for the cost of unnecessary medical services. *New England Journal of Medicine* 299 (13 July): 76-80.

Eisenberg, John M., and S. V. Williams. 1981. Cost containment and changing physicians' practice behavior: Can the fox learn to guard the chicken coop? *Journal of the American Medical Association* 246:2195-2201.

Emerson, Richard M. 1962. Power-dependence relations. *American Sociological Review* 27 (February): 31–41.

Enthoven, Alain. 1980. *Health plan: The only practical solution to the soaring cost of medical care.* Reading, Mass.: Addison-Wesley.

Etzioni, Amitai. 1974. Alternative conceptions of accountability. *Hospital Progress* 55 (June): 34–39.

Feldstein, Martin S. 1965. Hospital cost variation and case-mix differences. *Medical Care* 3:95–103.

Feldstein, Martin S., and J. Schuttinga. 1977. Hospital cost in Massachusetts: A methodological study. *Inquiry* 14:22–31.

Feldstein, Paul. 1968. An analysis of reimbursement plans. In *Reimbursement incentives for hospital and medical care: Objectives and alternatives.* Research Report 26. Washington, D.C.: Social Security Administration, Office of Research and Statistics.

Fineberg, Harvey. 1979. Gastric freezing: A study of diffusion of a medical innovation. National Academy of Sciences, Washington, D.C. Mimeographed.

Finkler, Stephen A. 1981. Flexible budgets: The next step in health care financial control. *Health Services Manager* 14 (May): 6–11.

Freidson, Eliot. 1970. *Professional dominance: The social structure of medical care.* Chicago: Atherton.

———. 1976. *Doctoring together.* New York: Elsevier.

Furst, Richard W., and Robert E. Markland. 1980. How hospital capital investment and operating costs relate. *Inquiry* 17:313–17.

Gabel, Jon R., and Alan C. Monheit. 1983. Will competition plans change insurer-provider relationships? *Milbank Memorial Fund Quarterly: Health and Society* 61:614–40.

Galbraith, Jay. 1973. *Designing complex organizations.* Reading, Mass.: Addison-Wesley.

Galbraith, John K. 1973. *Economics and the public purpose.* Boston: Houghton Mifflin.

Ginsburg, Paul B., and Frank A. Sloan. 1984. Hospital cost shifting. *New England Journal of Medicine* 310 (5 April): 893–98.

Ginzberg, Eli. 1983a. Cost containment—imaginary and real. *New England Journal of Medicine* 308 (19 May): 1220–24.

———. 1983b. The delivery of health care: What lies ahead. *Inquiry* 20:201–17.

Goldsmith, Jeff C. 1980. The health care market: Can hospitals survive? *Harvard Business Review* 58 (September–October): 100–112.

Gordon, Myron J., and Gordon Shillinglaw. 1974. *Accounting: A management approach.* Homewood, Ill.: Richard D. Irwin.

Gordon, Paul J. 1964. The top management triangle in the voluntary hospital. *Hospital Administration* 9 (Spring): 46–72.

Green, Stephen. 1975. Professional/bureaucratic conflict: The case of the medical profession in the National Health Service. *Sociology Review* 23 (February): 121–41.

Greer, Ann Lennarson. 1983. Medical conservatism and technological acquisitiveness: The paradox of hospital technology adoptions. Urban Research Center, University of Wisconsin, Milwaukee. Mimeographed.

Guest, Robert. 1972. The role of the doctor in institutional management. In *Organization research on health institutions,* ed. Basil Georgopoulos. Ann Arbor, Mich.: Institute for Social Research.
Hage, Jerold. 1974. *Communication and organizational control: Cybernetics in health and welfare settings.* New York: John Wiley.
Hamilton, Diane E., and Gilbey Kamens. 1979. A case study of prospective reimbursement in New York. Abt Associates Report no. 79-4(g) to Health Care Financing Administration.
Harris, Jeffrey E. 1977. The internal organization of hospitals: Some economic implications. *Bell Journal of Economics* 8 (Autumn): 467-82.
———. 1979. Regulation and internal control in hospitals. *Bulletin of the New York Academy of Medicine* 55 (January): 88-103.
Havighurst, Clark C. 1980. Antitrust enforcement in the medical services industry: What does it all mean? *Milbank Memorial Fund Quarterly* 58 (Winter): 89-124.
Hellinger, Fred J. 1979. Hospital rate-regulation programs and proposals: A survey and analysis. *Topics in Health Care Financing* 6 (Fall): 5-13.
———. 1982. Perspectives on Enthoven's consumer choice health plan. *Inquiry* 19:199-210.
Heyssel, Robert M., et al. 1984. Decentralized management in a teaching hospital. *New England Journal of Medicine* 310 (31 May): 1477-80.
Hickson, David J., et al. 1971. A strategic contingencies theory of intraorganizational power. *Administrative Science Quarterly* 16:216-29.
Hoey, J., et al. 1982. Physician sensitivity to the price of diagnostic tests: A U.S.-Canadian analysis. *Medical Care* 29:302-7.
Hughes, E. F. X., et al. 1978. *Cost containment programs: A policy analysis.* Cambridge, Mass.: Ballinger.
Iglehart, John. 1982. The new era of prospective payment for hospitals. *New England Journal of Medicine* 307 (11 November): 1288-92.
Institute of Medicine. 1976. *Assessing quality in health care: An evaluation.* Washington, D.C.: National Academy of Sciences.
Jacobs, Philip. 1974. A survey of economic models of hospitals. *Inquiry* 11:83-97.
Joskow, Paul L. 1981. *Controlling hospital costs: The role of government regulation.* Cambridge, Mass.: MIT Press.
Kane, Nancy. 1984. Analysis of financial capacity, capital needs, and service constituencies in New York City hospitals. Health Capital Project working paper, Harvard School of Public Health, Boston. Mimeographed.
Kaplan, S. X. 1980. Private sector shows how to cut health care costs. *HCFA Forum* 4:2-7.
Keith, Judith M. 1980. Anesthesiologist vs. administrator: A classic power struggle. In *Hospital administrator,* ed. James O. Hepner, pp. 303-6. Saint Louis: C. V. Mosby.
Kinzer, David M. 1980. Cost reductions remain goal of federal regs. *Hospitals* 54 (1 January): 91-94.
———. 1983. Massachusetts and California—two kinds of hospital cost control. *New England Journal of Medicine* 308 (7 April): 838-41.
Kleinberg, Warren M. 1980. Cost containment and ambulatory medicine. In *The*

physician and cost control, ed. Edward J. Carels, Duncan Neuhauser, and William B. Stason, pp. 53-62. Cambridge, Mass.: Oegeschlager, Gunn and Hain.

Kotelchuck, David. 1976. *Prognosis negative: crisis in the health care system.* New York: Vintage.

Krause, Elliott A. 1977. *Power and illness: The political sociology of health and medical care.* New York: Elsevier.

Lave, J. R., and L. B. Lave. 1971. The extent of role differentiation among hospitals. *Health Service Resource* 6:15-38.

Lave, J. R., L. B. Lave, and L. P. Silverman. 1972. Hospital cost estimation controlling for case-mix. *Applied Economics* 4:165-80.

Lave, J. R., and S. Reinhardt. 1976. The cost and length of a hospital stay. *Inquiry* 13:327-43.

La Violette, Suzanne. 1980. Snowed under by regs, hospitals unbundle services. *Modern Healthcare* 10 (December): 52-60.

Lawrence, Paul R., and Jay W. Lorsch. 1967. *Organization and environment.* Boston: Division of Research, Graduate School of Business Administration, Harvard University.

Lee, Maw Lin. 1971. A conspicuous production theory of hospital behavior. *Southern Economic Journal* 38 (July): 48-58.

Levi, Margaret. 1980. Functional redundancy and the process of professionalization: The case of registered nurses in the United States. *Journal of Health Politics, Policy and Law* 5 (Summer): 333-53.

Longo, Daniel R., and Gary A. Chase. 1984. Structural determinants of hospital closure. *Medical Care* 22 (May): 388-402.

McClelland, David C., and David G. Winter. 1969. *Motivating economic achievement.* New York: Free Press.

McClure, Walter. 1976. The medical care system under national health insurance: Four models. *Journal of Health Politics, Policy and Law* 1 (Spring): 21-68.

McGarrah, Robert E., Jr., et al. 1976. PSRO: Doctor accountability or consumer disaster? In *Prognosis negative: Crisis in the health care system,* ed. David Kotelchuck, pp. 404-13. New York: Vintage.

Mechanic, David. 1980. *Future issues in health care: Social policy and the rationing of medical services.* New York: Free Press.

―――. 1981. Some dilemmas in healthcare policy. *Milbank Memorial Fund Quarterly: Health and Society* 59:1-15.

―――. 1984. The transformation of health providers. *Health Affairs* 3 (Spring): 65-72.

Millman, Marcia. 1977. *The unkindest cut: Life in the backrooms of medicine.* New York: Morrow.

Monsma, George Jr. 1980. Marginal revenue and the demand for physicians' services. In *Empirical studies in health economics,* ed. Herbert Klarman. Baltimore: Johns Hopkins University Press.

Moore, Stephen H., et al. 1983. Does the primary care gatekeeper control the cost of healthcare? Lessons from the SAFECO experience. *New England Journal of Medicine* 309 (1 December): 1400-1404.

Neuhauser, Duncan. 1972. The hospital as a matrix organization. *Hospital Administration* 17 (Fall): 8-25.
Newhouse, Joseph. 1970. Toward a theory of nonprofit institutions: An economic model of a hospital. *American Economic Review* 60 (March): 64-74.
Newhouse, Joseph, et al. 1981. Some interim results from a controlled trial of cost sharing in health insurance. *New England Journal of Medicine* 305 (17 December): 1501-7.
Pauly, Mark V., and Michael Redisch. 1973. The not-for-profit hospital as a physician cooperative. *American Economic Review* 63 (March): 87-99.
Perrow, Charles. 1963. Goals and power structures. In *The hospital in modern society*, ed. Elliot Freidson. London: Free Press of Glencoe.
Pettigrew, Andrew W. 1973. *The politics of organizational decision-making*. London: Tavistock.
Platt, Roger. 1974. Cost containment — another view. *New England Journal of Medicine* 309 (22 September): 726-30.
Pondy, Louis R. 1970. Toward a theory of internal resource-allocation. In *Power in organizations*, ed. Mayer N. Zald, pp. 270-311. Nashville, Tenn.: Vanderbilt University Press.
Raffel, Marshall. 1984. *Comparative health systems*. University Park: Pennsylvania State University Press.
Redisch, Michael A. 1978. Physician involvement in hospital decision-making. In *Hospital cost containment: Selected notes for future policy*, ed. Michael Zubkoff, Ira E. Raskin, and Ruth S. Hanft, pp. 217-43. New York: Prodist.
Relman, Arnold S. 1980a. The allocation of medical resources by physicians. *Journal of Medical Education* 55:94-104.
———. 1980b. The new medical-industrial complex. *New England Journal of Medicine* 303 (23 October): 963-70.
Roemer, Milton, et al. 1975. Co-payments for ambulatory care: Penny-wise and pound-foolish. *Medical Care* 13 (June): 457-66.
Roos, Noralou P. 1974. Influencing the health care system: Policy alternatives. *Public Policy* 22 (Spring): 139-67.
Ruchlin, Hirsch S., and Harry M. Rosen. 1980. Short-run hospital responses to reimbursement rate changes. *Inquiry* 17:42-53.
Sahin, Kenan E., and Amy K. Taylor. 1979. Employer acquisition of health-care facilities: a possible outcome of escalating premiums? *Sloan Management Review* 20 (Summer): 61-75.
Salkever, David S., and Thomas W. Bice. 1978. Certificate of need legislation and hospital costs. In *Hospital cost containment: selected notes for future policy*, ed. Michael Zubkoff, Ira E. Raskin, and Ruth S. Hanft, pp. 429-60. New York: Prodist.
Saltman, Richard B., and David W. Young. 1981. The hospital power equilibrium: An alternative view of the cost containment dilemma. *Journal of Health Politics, Policy and Law* 6 (Fall): 391-418.
———. 1983. Hospital cost containment and the quest for institutional growth: A behavioral analysis. *Journal of Public Health Policy* 4:313-34.
Schlenker, Robert E., and Nancy H. Shanks. 1983. The private sector and compe-

tition in health care markets. *Journal of Health Politics, Policy and Law* 8 (Fall): 598–606.

Schroeder, Steven A. 1980. Variations in physician practice patterns: A review of medical cost implications. In *The physician and cost contorol,* ed. Edward J. Carels, Duncan Neuhauser, and William B. Stason, pp. 23–50. Cambridge, Mass.: Oegeschlager, Gunn and Hain.

Schroeder, Steven A., and J. A. Showstack. 1978. Financial incentives to perform medical procedures and laboratory tests: Illustrative models of office practice. *Medical Care* 16:289–98.

Schultz, Rockwell I., and Jerry Rose. 1973. Can hospitals be expected to control costs? *Inquiry* 10:3–8.

Seaver, Douglas J. 1977. Hospital revises role, reaches out to cultivate and capture markets. *Hospitals* 51 (1 June): 59–63.

Selznick, Philip. 1949. *TVA and the grassroots.* Berkeley: University of California Press.

Sigelman, Daniel W. 1983. Palm-reading the invisible hand: A critical examination of pro-competitive reform proposals. *Journal of Health Politics, Policy and Law* 6 (Winter): 578–620.

Silvers, J. B. 1981. Competitive economics of health care providers in the 1980s: The case of the large national clinics. Unpublished manuscript, Case Western Reserve University, Cleveland.

Simborg, Donald. 1981. DRG creep: A new hospital acquired disease. *New England Journal of Medicine* 304 (18 June): 1602–4.

Sloan, Frank A. 1983. Rate regulation as a strategy for hospital cost control: Evidence from the last decade. *Milbank Memorial Fund Quarterly: Health and Society* 61 (Spring): 195–221.

Smith, Harvey L. 1955. Two lines of authority: The hospital's dilemma. *Modern Hospital* 84 (March): 59–64.

Snoke, Albert W. 1982. What good is legislation – or planning – if we can't make it work? The need for a comprehensive approach to health and welfare. *American Journal of Public Health* 72 (September): 1028–33.

Soliman, Soliman Y., and W. L. Hughes. 1983. DRG payments and net contribution variance analysis. *Health Care Financial Management* 13 (October): 78–86.

Solomons, David. 1965. *Divisional performance: Measurement and control.* Homewood, Ill.: Dow Jones–Irwin.

Starr, Paul. 1980. Changing the balance of power in American medicine. *Milbank Memorial Fund Quarterly* 58 (Winter): 166–72.

———. 1982. *The social transformation of American medicine.* New York: Basic Books.

Stern, R. S., and A. M. Epstein. 1985. Institutional responses to prospective payment based on Diagnosis-Related Groups: Implications for cost quality and access. *New England Journal of Medicine* 312:621–27.

Stockman, David A. 1981. Premises for a medical marketplace: A neoconservative's vision of how to transform the health system. *Health Affairs* 1 (Winter): 5–18.

Stone, Deborah A. 1980a. *The limits of professional power: National health care in the Federal Republic of Germany.* Chicago: University of Chicago Press.
———. 1980b. The problem of monopoly power in federal health policy. *Milbank Memorial Fund Quarterly* 58 (Winter): 50–53.
Taylor, Humphrey, and Asha Paranjpe. 1984. *The Equitable healthcare survey II: Physicians' attitudes toward cost containment.* New York: Equitable Life Assurance Society of the United States.
Thompson, J. D., R. B. Fetter, and C. D. Mross. 1975. Case mix and resource use. *Inquiry* 12:300–312.
Todd, Hamilton Smith, Jr., and Stephen Charles Rice. 1979. *Costs and decision-making processes in non-profit, general purpose hospitals.* Springfield, Va.: National Technical Information Service.
Unger, Walter. 1982. California charts a new competitive course. *Healthcare Financial Management* 36:60–74.
Vancil, Richard F. 1973. What kind of management control do you need? *Harvard Business Review* 51 (March–April): 75–86.
Vancil, Richard F., and Peter Lorange. 1975. Strategic planning in diversified companies. *Harvard Business Review* 53 (January–February): 81–90.
Warner, Kenneth E. 1978. Effects of hospital cost containment on the development and use of medical technology. *Milbank Memorial Fund Quarterly* 56 (Spring): 187–211.
Weiblen, Jack W. 1980. Maintaining cost-saving incentives in physician contracts. In *Hospital administrator,* ed. James O. Hepner, pp. 287–90. Saint Louis: C. V. Mosby.
Weiner, Stephen M. 1977. "Reasonable cost" reimbursement for inpatient hospital services under Medicare and Medicaid: The emergence of public control. *American Journal of Law and Medicine* 3 (Spring): 1–47.
Weller, Geoffrey R., and Pranlal Manga. 1983. The push for reprivatization of health care services in Canada, Britain, and the United States. *Journal of Health Politics, Policy and Law* 8 (Fall): 495–518.
Wennberg, John E. 1977. Change in tonsillectomy rates. *Pediatrics* 59:821.
Wood, Charles T. 1982. Relate hospital charges to use of services. *Harvard Busi-Business Review* 60 (March–April): 123–30.
Worthington, Paul N. 1976. Prospective reimbursement of hospitals to promote efficiency: New Jersey. *Inquiry* 13:302–8.
Young, David W. 1979a. Administrative theory and administrative systems: A synthesis among diverging fields of inquiry. *Accounting Organizations and Society* 4:235–44.
———. 1979b. *The managerial process in human service agencies.* New York: Praeger.
———. 1981. The role of transfer prices in the purchase of service systems. In *Organization and the human services: Cross-disciplinary reflections,* ed. Herman D. Stein, pp. 233–44. Philadelphia: Temple University Press.
———. 1982. Nonprofits need surplus, too. *Harvard Business Review* 60 (January–February): 124–31.
———. 1984. *Financial control in health care.* Homewood, Ill.: Dow Jones-Irwin.

Young, David W., and Nancy M. Kane. 1984. Capital distribution in health care: The need for a visible hand. Health Capital Project working paper, Harvard School of Public Health, Boston. Mimeographed.

Young, David W., and Richard B. Saltman. 1982. Medical practice, case mix, and cost containment: A new role for the physician. *Journal of the American Medical Association* 287 (12 February): 801–5.

———. 1983a. Preventive medicine for hospital costs. *Harvard Business Review* 61 (January–February): 126–33.

———. 1983b. Prospective reimbursement and the hospital power equilibrium: A matrix-based management control system. *Inquiry* 20:20–33.

Zuidema, George D. 1980. The problem of cost containment in teaching hospitals: The Johns Hopkins experience. *Surgery* 87 (January): 41–44.

Index

Andrews, K. R., 161
Anthony, R. N., 145, 153, 155, 180, 181, 182, 183
Ashkenas, R., 177
Atkinson, J. G., 14
Authority structure, for hospital control system, 161

Badgley, R. F., 7
Barer, M. L., 7
Barnard, C. I., 161, 182
Barnes, L. B., 25
Bauer, K. G., 15, 175
Bauerschmidt, A. D., 182
Beck, R. G., 7
Bedford, N. M., 180, 182
Begley, C. E., 180
Behavioral incentives, implications for cost containment, 52-53
Bernard, C., 179
Bice, T. W., 15, 178, 180
Biles, B., 14
Blishen, B. R., 30, 34, 178
Blumenthal, D., 1
Borgenhammer, E., 175
Boston Consulting Group, 150
Bower, J. L., 25, 182
Brady, J. F., 176
Brook, R. H., 6
Brown, J. B., 47, 177, 178, 180
Brown, L. D., 8, 175
Buchanan, J. M., 23
Bucher, R., 176
Budgeting, 147
Butler, R. J., 25

Canadian experience, 176
Caper, P., 1
Capital budgeting process, comparison between the two hospitals, 134-36
Capital costs, vicious cycle of, 137
Carels, E. J., 175
Carnoy, J., 183
Case mix, 13
Case studies, theoretical implications of, 121
Chandler, A. D., 181
Charns, M. P., 182

Chase, G. A., 10
Chicago *Tribune,* 10
Christenson, C. J., 179
Clarkson, K., 23
Clinical treatment protocols, 167-68
Coffee, L., 183
Cohodes, D. R., 10, 181
Congressional Budget Office, 15
Conrad, D., 6, 7, 11, 175
Copayments, 4-9
Coser, R. L., 28, 29
Cost accounting structure, for matrix-based control system, 170
Cost containment: issues, comparison between the two hospitals, 129-38; and management control systems, 144-47
Cost sharing, 4-12; and hospital-based programs, 143-44, 175
Cost-influencing variables, 155; and their controling forces, 159-60
Croog, S. J., 176
Crozier, M., 21, 25-38, 53, 135
Curran, W. J., 177
Cyert, R. M., 25, 182

Dalton, G. W., 25
Davis, K., 16
Davis, S., 162, 182
Dearden, J., 180, 182
Deductibles, 4-9
Densen, P. M., 175
Detsky, A. S., 175
Diagnosis-related groups, 2, 16, 17, 36, 129-31, 169; and cost-influencing variables, 154-56
Dolan, A. K., 43
Doremus, H. D., 181
Dowling, W. L., 14, 181
Dowries: and the capital budgeting process, 134; and prestige, 130, 180; role of, 125, 129-31
DRGs. *See* Diagnosis-related groups

Egdahl, R. H., 8
Eisenberg, J. M., 169
Emerson, R. M., 25
Enthoven, A., 10, 11
Epstein, A. M., 175, 181

195

Index

Etzioni, A., 22, 23
Evaluation, 147
Exchange model, 21

Fairness and goal congruence, absence of, in existing reimbursement systems, 156-57; defined, 181
Feldstein, M. S., 159, 175
Feldstein, P., 151
Fetter, R. B., 175
Fineberg, H., 45, 165
Finkler, S. A., 181
Freidson, E., 30, 177
Freyer, R., 178
Furst, R. W., 180

Gabel, J. R., 7, 8, 12
Galbraith, J. K., 40, 41, 43, 47
Galbraith, Jay, 182
Gellhorn, A., 177
Ginsburg, P. B., 52
Ginzberg, E., 7, 175
Goal congruence. *See* Fairness and goal congruence
Goldsmith, J. C., 15, 16, 178
Gordon, M. J., 183
Gordon, P. J., 176
Green, S., 176
Greer, A. L., 144, 165
Growth. *See* Institutional growth
Guest, R., 29

Hage, J., 25
Hamilton, D. E., 175, 178
Harris, J. E., 23, 32, 34, 47, 177, 182
Havighurst, C., 29, 175
Health care expenditures, 4
Health maintenance organizations, 10, 11, 16, 43
Health policy and management, implications of findings for, 138-40
Hegarty, S., 176
Hellinger, F. J., 15, 175
Heyssel, R. M., 182
Hickson, D. J., 25
HMOs. *See* Health maintenance organizations
Hoey, J., 169
Hospitals: cost behavior, 151; financial pressure on, 175; occupational strategies in, 28; parallels with Crozier's industrial monopoly, 32; physicians' effort to influence decision making, 29; power equilibrium, motives in group strategies, 39; power equilibrium theory, likely validity of, 122; theories of decision making, 21; top management, 169-72
Hughes, E.F.X., 15
Hughes, W. L., 183
Human Relations School, 182

Iglehardt, J., 1, 36
Incentives: behavioral (*see* Behavioral incentives); consequences of group behavioral, 49; for administrators, 46-48, 178; for other occupational groups, 48-49; for physicians, 42-46
Infant mortality rates, 175
Institute of Medicine, 15
Institutional comparisons, Oak Memorial vs. Peninsula, 123, 128-29
Institutional growth: empirical findings, 128; and hospital administrators, 46-48; impetus toward, 39, 40-41

Jacobs, P., 21, 22
Joskow, P. L., 175

Kamens, G., 175, 178
Kane, N., 10, 181
Kaplan, S. X., 175
Keith, J. M., 176
Kinzer, D. M., 1, 35
Kleinberg, W. M., 175
Koo, L., 183
Kotelchuck, D., 177
Krause, E. A., 30, 34, 178

Lave, J. R., 159, 175
Lave, L. B., 159, 175
LaViolette, S., 178
Lawrence, P. R., 39, 40, 161, 162, 182
Lee, M. L., 23, 29, 178
Levi, M., 178
Liaison Committee on Graduate Medical Education, 179
Liaison Committee on Medical Education, 179
Lindsey, C. M., 23
Longo, D. R., 10
Lorange, P., 164, 182
Lorsch, J. W., 29, 40, 161, 182

McClelland, D. C., 25
McClure, W., 47, 178
McCullough, A. E., 25
McGarrah, R. E., 15
Management control: principles, absence of, in existing reimbursement systems, 153–56; process, 145, 146, 163–67; structure, 145, 146, 158–63
Management control systems: centralized versus decentralized, 147, 148; and cost containment, 144, 147
Management responsibility system, realigned, 171
Manga, P., 6, 8
March, J. G., 25, 182
Market-based proposals, implications of, 3–12; for patients, 6; for providers, 9
Market misconception, 17
Markland, R. E., 180
Marks, H. M., 47, 177, 180
Marmor, T. R., 6, 7, 11, 175
Matrix-based control system, 167, 170; advantages of, 172
Matrix-based managerial approach, 163
Matrix theory, 162
Mayo, E., 182
Measurement, 147
Mechanic, D., 7, 12, 46, 47, 177
Medical submarkets, 18
Methodological questions, 120–21
Millman, M., 29, 33, 45, 176
Monheit, A. C., 7, 8, 12
Monsma, G., 44, 45, 177
Moore, S. H., 8, 12
Mross, C. D., 175

Neuhauser, D., 162
Newhouse, J., 6, 7, 23
Nurses, unionization of, 178

Oak Memorial Medical Center: administration, perceptions of, 110–12; attending physician/house officers, interaction of, 85; budget structure of, 73; dowries, 106–9; dowries, chiefs' view of, 112–14; financial incentives, 76; fiscal affairs, role of, 117–19; full-salaried/part-time physicians, interaction, 84; interactions among service chiefs, 80; interactions between medical and support staff, 86; interactions between physicians and administrators, 73–78; interactions within services, 81; interactions within the administration, 78–79; interactions within the medical staff, 79–86; middle management perspective on program decision making, 105–9; organizational chart, 74; outpatient psychiatry, 180; practice funds, 77; prestige incentives, 75; resource allocation criteria, 114–15; resource-influencing techniques, 116–17; senior management perspective on program decision making, 104–5; service chief on program decision making, 110–17; the setting, 72
Operating activities, 166–67
Operating control, centralized, 152
Operating decisions, 150–53
Organism model, 21
Other occupational group strategies, empirical findings, 126–27

Paranjpe, A., 12, 16
Patient dumping, 10
Pauly, M. V., 23, 30
Peer pressure, informal mechanisms, 43
Peninsula Community Hospital: anesthesia department of, 100; budget structure, 59; capital equipment, 101–2; emergency room, 99; endoscopy suite, 96–98; inpatient dialysis service, 93; interactions between medical and support staff, 65–67; interactions between physicians and administration, 59–63; interactions within the medical staff, 63–65; medical staff cost containment issues, 67–71; midwife program, 98; new services, 92–98; organization chart, 58; outpatient psychiatry clinic, 92; program initiatives, 92–103; programmatic decision-making criteria, 89–92; renovations, 102–3; reorganization of existing services, 98–101; the setting, 57; sports medicine, 94; telemetry unit, 94–96
Perrow, C., 22
Pettigrew, A., 25
Physicians: control over quality, 177; financial influences, 44; incentives in decision making, 177; influence upon hospital decision making, 49–51, 176; integration into hospital management, 167; and market-oriented proposals, 11–12; motivation of, 125–26; peer monitoring among, 171; personal influences, 45;

Physicians, *continued*
  practice characteristics, 179; professional influences, 42; strategies between, empirical findings, 127-28; variance in practice styles of, 178
Platt, R., 17
Policymakers, challenge to, 19
Pondy, L. R., 23
Power and conflict, model of, 25
Power equilibrium and cost containment, 35; theory of, 25-38
Power relationship between administrators and physicians, 122-25, 180
Prestige, importance of, 47, 122-26
Program development process, the, 131-34
Programming, 163-66; decisions, 147-50
Program proliferation, 146, 149
Programs, and health system actors, 132
Prospective reimbursement program, defined, 181

Raffel, M., 175, 176
Rand Corporation study, 6, 7
Rate-setting perspective, 14
Redisch, M. A., 23, 29, 30, 33, 45, 176, 177
Reece, J. S., 182
Regulation, failure of, 13
Reimbursement systems, structural failures of, 153-57
Reinhardt, S., 159
Relman, A. S., 165, 169, 177
Reporting, 147
Revenue and cost considerations, 136-38
Rice, S. C., 23
Roemer, M., 6, 7
Roemer's law, 45
Roethlisberger, F., 182
Roos, N. P., 23
Rose, J., 46, 178
Rosen, H. M., 14, 16
Rosoff, A. J., 169
Ruchlin, H. S., 14, 16

SAFECO, 8, 12
Sahin, K. E., 175
Salkever, D. S., 15, 178, 180
Saltman, R. B., 160, 172, 178, 181, 182
Schlenker, R. E., 175
Schramm, C. J., 14
Schroeder, S. A., 18, 44, 45, 177
Schultz, R. I., 46, 178
Schuttinga, J., 159

Seaver, D. J., 178
Selznick, P., 173
Shanks, N. H., 175
Shillinglaw, G., 183
Shoeman, M., 180
Showstack, J. A., 45
Sigelman, D. W., 12, 175
Silverman, L. P., 175
Silvers, J. B., 178
Simborg, D., 16
Sloan, F. A., 15, 16, 52
Smith, H. L., 23
Smith, R. D., 7
Snoke, A. W., 8, 12
Sociological models, 30
Soliman, S. Y., 183
Solomons, D., 180
Starr, P., 176, 178
Stelling, J., 176
Stern, R. S., 175, 181
Stockman, D. A., 4
Stone, D. A., 169, 176

Taylor, A. K., 175
Taylor, H., 12, 16
Thompson, J. D., 175
Todd, H. S., 23
Traxler, H., 180

Unger, W., 36

Vancil, R. F., 153, 155, 156, 164, 181, 182
Variance analysis, structure of, 172
Variance-based reporting system, 171
Ver Steeg, D. F., 176

Warner, K. E., 29, 32
Weiblen, J. W., 176
Weiner, S. M., 175
Weisbord, M., 182
Weller, G. R., 6, 8
Welsch, G. A., 183
Wennberg, J. E., 45, 159
Williams, S. V., 169
Winter, D. G., 25
Wood, C. T., 183
Worthington, P. N., 175

Young, D. W., 153, 160, 172, 177, 178, 179, 181, 182

Zalesnick, A., 25
Zuidema, G. D., 182

David W. Young, formerly associate professor of management at the Harvard School of Public Health, is professor of accounting and control in the School of Management at Boston University. His most recent book is *Financial Control in Health Care.*
Richard B. Saltman, formerly a research associate in political science at the Harvard School of Public Health, is associate professor in the School of Public Health at the University of Massachusetts at Amherst. He is currently conducting comparative research on hospital and physician behavior in Scandinavia.

The Johns Hopkins University Press

The Hospital Power Equilibrium

This book was composed in English Times text and display type by Capitol Communication Systems from a design by Chris L. Smith. It was printed on 50-lb. Sebago Eggshell Cream paper and bound in Kivar 5 by Bookcrafters.